Discover How A Cocktail of Simple Molecules Can Prevent and Fight Cancer and Other Diseases

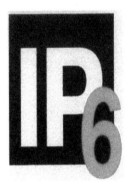

+

Inositol

NATURE'S MEDICINE FOR THE MILLENNIUM

PROF ABULKALAM M. SHAMSUDDIN, MD, PhD

IP-6 RESEARCH
BALTIMORE
U.S.A.
www.ip-6.net

ISBN: 978-984-33-2708-6

First printing: February 2011

Printed in the United States of America

Available from Amazon.com and other fine retailers

US$ 19.97

To my Dad and my uncle, Subid, Mary-Claire and other uncountable millions of victims of cancer...

May this humble effort help reduce human suffering

iv

TABLE OF CONTENTS

Page

PREFACE

Dad had a holistic approach to healing, a concept though becoming fashionable now, was quite unorthodox at the time (the 1950's and 60's). Dad wanted me to be a physician like him perhaps with the secret desire that I could take over his practice so that he could retire, hangout with his buddies and be proud of his son though Dad was never the bragging type. But his son had no intention of being a physician [I wanted to be a physicist]. At the end, Dad had his way, so I had to go to medical school, quite reluctantly though.

During my first year of medical school at the University of Dhaka, one of my most favorite uncles – my mother's brother was diagnosed with small cell (oat cell) cancer of the lung. We were told to take him home so that he could die with dignity, in about 6 weeks! And he did. That was my first close encounter with cancer. It would have been an interesting story if I said that, that's what motivated me to go into cancer research; but it was not.

The first year was boring as we were learning only anatomy and histology by pure memorization. I tried hard in vain to get into trouble so that I could be kicked out of medical school. In those days in my medical school, the students, no matter how brilliant they were could be in deep trouble, especially if they were men, a sort of reverse gender discrimination, for challenging professors, even the lowest ranking instructors! Coupled with the inspiration by Professor Abdur Rahman of Physiology, the subjects in second year were interesting enough for me to give-up the idea of my being a physicist. In the third year (5 years of total schooling) we started learning about cancer and tumor immunity and I found the subject fascinating. The choice was made. The irony is Dad too passed away with the same "oat cell" (small cell) cancer of the lung as my uncle did, only a year before I started my research in cancer. He too had only a few days to live after the diagnosis. The scourge has affected two of my dearest friends; Subid lost the battle, while true to her character, Mary-Claire has been successfully fighting it, thus far.

Aside from my parents, I have been most fortunate to have some of the best people as my teachers (e.g. Professor Abdur Rahman) and mentors. The late Dr Benjamin F. Trump, then the Chair of Pathology at the University of Maryland, School of Medicine in Baltimore gave me the opportunity and guidance in my career in cancer research, for which I am indebted to him. He was an iconoclast and was quite supportive of me being one.

The tragic and untimely death of my favorite uncle and my Dad left me ponder: by the time a cancer is diagnosed, it's too late. What if they could be diagnosed early on? What if there was some way to even prevent this from happening? Thus, beginning 1975, at the University of Maryland, I started my studies of cancer with the approach of early detection and prevention; that we need screening tests for cancers so that they can be detected at very early stages (even before a cancer has formed) and then prophylactic measures taken so that they can be nipped at the bud.

Professor Trump had essentially built an empire of cancer research where almost every major type of cancer was being investigated. I had found the cancer of kidney interesting and expressed my desire to work on it; but that was taken – several people were working on it. What was not popular (for obvious aesthetic reason) was the colon project. And that's what I was assigned to.

As I started to study the subject, I was astonished by the extreme dogmatism – the overwhelming majority of publications cried (and still do) that all colon cancers come from some drumstick shaped benign growths called polyps! And then there were a very small minority, albeit rather distinguished pathologists of the era who stated the contrary – colon cancers arise *de novo* (anew) and not from the polyps! Notwithstanding the quantity of papers on one side and the quality of pathologist on the other, I found them both illogical. So, I set out to find the truth myself with much humility.

Though many before me had studied the normal histology and anatomy of colon and rectum, I wanted to learn them the hard way, by myself and learn what really is normal, for only then I would be able to recognize the abnormal, especially if they are subtle. Of course, Professor Trump was ecstatic. Now, since we use rats and mice in routine experiments and then extrapolate the data to the human, my approach was to study the normal colons of rats, mice and humans. While the former two are easy to study, how can we be absolutely sure that the human colon one is looking at is perfectly normal? In other words, if one takes the colon from a surgical specimen containing colon cancer or an autopsy of a patient dying of colon or other diseases, are their colons really normal?

Fortunately, a part of Dr Trump's cancer research 'empire' included 'Immediate Autopsy' program. According to the laws of the State of Maryland as in most states, all victims of accidental death undergo autopsy by the medical examiner (coroner). Since the medical examiner's office was affiliated with the University, the program allowed us pathologists to perform autopsy within minutes after a patient has been declared brain-dead. Most of these victims were rather young without any other diseases and since the specimens were obtained immediately after their death, the acquired tissues were in the best preserved form (the enzymes in the body run-a-mock after death and rapidly start to digest the cells and tissues). Since there is no way to predict when a patient would be pronounced brain-dead, much less when a patient will arrive, we had teams of pathologists and other scientists who were on-call 24 hours a day and 7 days a week. Each team had several members of the organ/tissue collection personnel – one each for lungs, liver, colon, pancreas, prostate, kidney, breast, etc., and then one person for electron microscopy and one pathologist to perform the autopsy – all carrying beepers. As luck would have it, almost always these Immediate Autopsies would take place in the dead of the night (a friend and colleague of mine from Israel, Dr. Rafaelle David was caught speeding while he was coming to collect his specimens one night at around 2 AM and got away by mentioning Dr. Trump and his Immediate autopsy program!). Owing to my vested personal interest, and being both a pathologist as well as a colon cancer researcher, I volunteered for much of the year. Colorectal samples obtained from these individuals served as *my* normal control human against which I compared the so-called "normal" that many before me had studied.

Based on this approach of investigation, I developed the "field-effect" concept of cancer formation in the colon. I showed that the cancer in colon can develop from the polyps as well as directly (*de novo*); some large studies suggest that as much as 80% of the colon cancers arise without going through the polyp! I also identified a subtle change in the mucus of the colon in non-cancerous areas. Exploiting this "field-effect" phenomenon and the marker galactose-galactosamine (Gal-GalNAc), my humble efforts resulted in invention of a very simple screening test for cancers of the colorectum. The same concept and the marker are operational in other cancers such as those of the lungs, breast, prostate, pancreas etc. Thus, I have presented these early detection strategies at the beginning of the book, in Chapter 1.

So, what does one do if a cancer is detected early, even before there is full-blown disease? Take preventive measures, of course! Quite coincidentally, around the time of development of cancer screening tests, I started to work on cancer preventive agents – the B-vitamin inositol and its parent molecule inositol hexaphosphate (IP$_6$), naturally abundant in cereals and legumes. Though IP$_6$ has been considered an anti-nutrient for a very, very long time, I decided to conduct experiments; the results showed that IP$_6$+Inositol have consistent and reproducible anti-cancer action (both preventive and therapeutic) against a wide range of tumors, a broad-spectrum anti-cancer cocktail.

It has been over a quarter of a century since I had first demonstrated the anti-cancer action of IP$_6$ and Inositol in the mid 1980's. As exciting as the anti-cancer function of this cocktail is, there are other actions which may have equal if not more benefits. One of the most significant is the effect on bone and dental health. Osteoporosis is an extremely common condition that debilitates people worldwide; it has been estimated to afflict 1 in 3 women and 1 in 12 men over the age of 50 throughout our planet. Having learnt from our cancer experiments that IP$_6$ & Inositol have the anti-proliferative and pro-differentiating (taming cells to behave in a normal and mature manner) function, I wanted to test what IP$_6$ & Inositol will do to the bone-forming and bone-destroying cells. Fascinatingly, IP$_6$ & Inositol stimulate the bone-forming cells and suppresses the bone destroying cells! This is not a trivial matter given the impact of osteoporosis to our seniors globally.

And that's not all. IP_6+Inositol also have other health benefits. Related to the subject of bone health is the dental health. I shall present evidence how IP_6+Inositol can protect our teeth from the damaging effect of soft-drinks and sports drinks. Work mostly from the laboratory of Professor Fèlix Grases in Spain show that IP_6 prevents stone formation in the kidney and other places. And there are additional health benefits in Alzheimer's disease, diabetes, cardiovascular diseases, immunity etc.

The book is neither meant to give advice on cancer treatment or medicine in general, conventional or alternative, nor should it be so considered. I am a pathologist and not an oncologist; my research has been focused on the Gal-GalNAc cancer screening test and IP_6/Inositol; thus, I shall restrict my comments only on these.

Anticipating that the book will be read by people with a wide-range of scientific knowledge and background, and not wishing to offend the highly informed readers, I have purposefully kept lot of things very simple. On the other-hand, to satisfy the curiosity of the inquisitives, and to remain credible, I have presented I believe just enough scientific information; those who find these unintelligible, should skip the sections, and move on to the next.

AbulKalam M. Shamsuddin

CHAPTER 1

EARLY DETECTION OF CANCER

Fundamental to the success of prevention programs of any disease is the detection of the problems. It includes identification of the people with existing disease and those who are at risk of developing the disease. Since my efforts in search of better health have been studying cancer, I shall focus on early detection of cancer only. Identification of people with cancer is relatively simple for most cancers because of symptoms from the disease; the individual, now a patient seeks medical attention.

Extensive work-up including a battery of diagnostic tests are performed and appropriate therapy is administered; regrettably, it is usually too late for many, if not for most as it does not prevent the disease. Hence the adage: an ounce of prevention is better than a pound of cure.

For an effective prevention program, we must actively seek individuals with cancer or high risk thereof from an apparently healthy non-compliant population. This is done by separating (i.e. screening) individuals into groups with high and low probability of cancer with the help of *rapid*, *simple* and *inexpensive* tests (screening tests). Implicit in the definition of screening is a promise that there is a benefit for those who participate; they will be followed with further diagnostic tests and future management of the problem. But you must keep in mind that a *screening test is never intended to give the full diagnosis*; hence the distinction from diagnostic tests. An individual who is screening test positive will need to undergo diagnostic procedures to confirm the presence of the disease.

Ideal screening tests should have a high sensitivity (proportion of diseased subjects who are test-positive) and specificity (proportion of non-diseased subjects who are test-negative), be simple and non-invasive or minimally invasive, easy to administer – therefore enjoying a high acceptability amongst populations and of course cost-effective. It would not be successful if it is shunned for discomfort, cultural, religious or other reasons.

Colorectal Cancer Screening

Colorectal cancer is the commonest cancer in the industrialized world. It has been estimated that without screening, a 50-year-old person at average risk has approximately a 530-in-10,000 chance of developing invasive cancer during the rest of his or her life. To that effect, a host of tests are used and/or recommended. The common ones are the fecal occult blood tests (FOBT), barium enema, X-rays and endoscopic visualization (colonoscopy, sigmoidoscopy etc.). The cost-effectiveness of these varies tremendously, thus their usefulness as screening assays are seriously in question. The high accuracy of barium enema and endoscopies are marred by their high cost and subject discomfort. On one hand, FOBTs are relatively cheap compared to the cost of barium enema and colonoscopy. On the other hand, while FOBTs are inexpensive, they are notoriously inaccurate and thus not cost-effective in the long run.

The then U.S. Congressional Office of Technology Assessment[1] estimated that by merely increasing the sensitivity of FOBT from 25% to 40%, the cost per year of life gained could be reduced by nearly 20%. Thus, if we use better screening tools, we would reduce the number of unnecessary diagnostic tests (colonoscopies) thereby decreasing the total national healthcare cost to the society (please see Table 1).

Table 1-1

Screening Regimen	Cost/yr of life gained from FOBT With 25% Sensitivity	Cost/yr of life gained from FOBT With 40% Sensitivity	$ Saving (%)
FOBT only	$43,167	$35,054	$8,113 (19%)
FOBT + Sigmoid[a]	$48,338	$42,509	$5,829 (12%)

Adapted from Congressional Office of Technology Assessment 1990;
[a]Sigmoidoscopy every 5 years

A simple fact is that the test looks for blood in stool as a surrogate for cancer; not only not all cancers

---

[1] US Congressional Office of Technology Assessment was established in 1972 and calling it an "unnecessary agency" closed on 29 September, 1995 as a cost-cutting measure.

do not bleed, but also not all bleedings are due to cancer; thus, the reason for their inaccuracy. On the other hand, the high accuracy of barium enema and colonoscopy are marred by their high cost and

> *"Occult blood testing is, at best an imperfect approach to the screening of colorectal cancer" –D. A. Ahlquist, Cancer volume 70: 1259-1265, 1992*

subject discomfort [ask any senior citizen who has been undergoing these!]. Notwithstanding the strong and persistent recommendation of radiologists and gastroenterologists [politics of medical economics?], these two *diagnostic assays do not fit the criteria of screening tests*.

The current trend to look for and remove any polyp by colonoscopy is also based on a faulty premise – in a 1975 paper that became most influential, Dr. Muto and co-workers merely reported the presence of cancer on polyps and concluded without scientific evidence that most colorectal cancers arise from polyps. Let's look at what Muto *et al* had stated (*Cancer* volume 36:2251-2270, 1975):

> *"...the majority of adenomas [polyps] do <u>not</u> become cancerous during a normal*

> *adult life span [underline mine]. The slow
> evolution of the polyp cancer sequence is
> stressed."*

Indeed Figure 9 of their 1975 *Cancer* paper shows
the life history of 10 villous polyps [who have the
highest potential of all polyps to become cancer-
ous], "selected because they illustrate how *these
tumors can remain benign over a long period of
time*, although 2 eventually became malignant…In
Case 8 the polyp-cancer sequence took at least 28
years;" (bold and italics mine) *8 of those 10 (80%)
villous polyps did not become malignant for at
least 22.5 years!*

Another paper, in the journal *Diseases of Colon
and Rectum* by S. Kozuka *et al* also published in
the same year (1975), as the oft-quoted Muto paper
albeit not as famous, reported that the usual time
for the polyps to become malignant [if and when]
is 18 years! Thus, these two papers clearly show
the long time for the polyps to become cancer if
they ever do. Supporting the strategy of prophylactic polypectomy, in 1993 Dr Winawer and colleagues claim to have reduced the incidence of colorectal cancer by colonoscopic polypectomy (*New
England Journal of Medicine* 329: 1977-1981).

But think for a moment! How an average follow-up period of merely 5.9 years could be sufficient to accurately evaluate the success of preventing polyp → cancer when the time-span is at least 3-4 times as long (Kozuka *et al* 1975, Muto *et al* 1975)?!

Now combine that with the following:

Dr. T. Shimoda *et al* have shown that the majority (~80%) of the cancers of the colon and rectum arise directly from the flat non-polypoid mucosa (not from the polyps)! Though this paper too was published in the journal *Cancer* (volume 64: 1138-1146, 1989), the medical community apparently did not learn from its teachings. This is not a trivial matter for, *if* the majority of colon cancers do not arise from the benign polyps, then why are we subjecting the entire populations to the horrible experience of routine colonoscopic examination at an extremely high cost to the society?

The other just as important if not more significant question is: if most colon cancers do not arise from the polyps but from the flat non-polypoid mucosa (as shown by Prof Shimoda *et al* and others, including experimental and clinical data from my lab), then how do we detect them? Clearly, by removing the polyps we may enjoy a false sense of security.

These are the questions that had guided me to perform experiments culminating in the development of a test for screening cancers of the colorectum which has also found its utility in other cancers as well.

Lessons from Rats and Mice:

I had conducted experiments with rats and mice to see how colon cancer forms in them, the earliest recognizable changes – both by microscope and by histochemical methods. I also grew colon tissue from rats and human in the Petri dishes in lab and exposed them to cancer-causing chemicals (carcinogens) and strived to learn from them as well, and see if I could make any correlation with the *in vivo* animal models and human disease. Also as a trained human pathologist, I then examined what the human colon near and far from the cancer looked like.

I learnt that the microscopic and histochemical changes in the human colon away from cancer are identical to those seen in the colons of rats treated

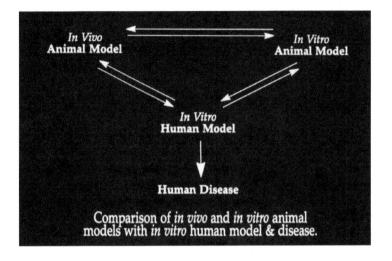

Comparison of *in vivo* and *in vitro* animal models with *in vitro* human model & disease.

with the carcinogen either *in vivo* (intact animals or *in vitro* (in Petri dishes); these changes are therefore the early evidence (or markers) of cancer formation. I reasoned that as a result of the generalized effect of the carcinogen throughout the entire field of the target tissue (in the colon and rectum the carcinogen arrives *via* blood supply or in feces); it is most likely that the tissue away from an obvious cancer would be abnormal. Thus, a rectal mucus sample should predict the presence or absence of a cancer in the colon.

The Rectal Mucus Test for Colorectal Cancer Screening

What's being assayed in the rectal mucus? The test looks for an abnormal sugar marker in the rectal mucin (not tissue) obtained during routine digital examination [that health care personnel should be performing on all patients routinely, anyway]. In normal individuals with healthy colon, the sugar is masked; in cancerous or pre-cancerous conditions and lesions it is unmasked to allow oxidation by an enzyme and finally visualized by a color reaction: a magenta color is positive whereas no color denotes a negative test result.

The test process is minimally invasive. The actual test is performed on a special paper which is storage stable for months, enabling the test strip to be mailed and processed in a central laboratory if so desired. It is reacted with an enzyme for 10 minutes, rinsed, reacted with a dye for 1 minute and rinsed again to read the color reaction. That's how simple it is! From a practical point of view, the tests, not just for colon cancer, but those for lung, breast etc. can be administered in doctors' office and have the results in 15 minutes or so, before you leave!

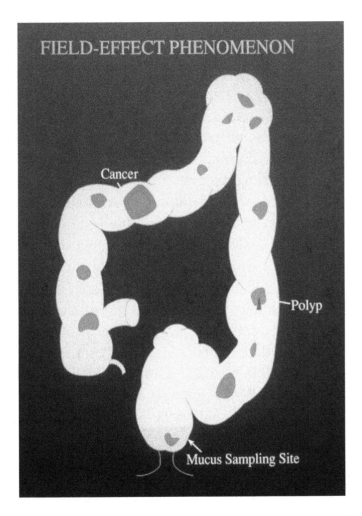

Figure 1-1: The "field-effect" phenomenon indicates that the entire field bears the brunt of the carcinogenic assault and express variable changes throughout. Rectum being a part of the large intestinal "field" and a sampling site is therefore likely to show the same changes.

How Good is the Rectal Mucus Test for Colorectal Cancer?

The pilot study of the test showed excellent result, all 13 patients with cancer scored positive (100% sensitivity) and so were only 4 of 58 asymptomatic otherwise normal individuals (54/58 = 93% specificity). Since reporting the results in the US-Canadian Academy of Pathology Annual Meeting in Chicago in March 1987 and the publication of the paper in 1988 (*Human Pathology* volume 19: pages 7-10) various investigators throughout the world evaluated the sensitivity and specificity of the test, variously called: the rectal mucus or the rectal mucin test (RMT), galactose oxidase test, galactose oxidase Schiff test (GOS Test) or Shams' test. The sample size and sample selection varied widely. Carefully designed studies with large sample size showed a sensitivity of 80% - 100% and specificity of 92% - 100%. The number of subjects in these clinical trials totals over 10,000; in the largest test, 6,480 patients were screened using this test in China. The results demonstrated a sensitivity of 94.4% and a specificity of 98.23 %. The test has been in use in China since the early 1990's.

Published in 2001, another clinical trial was performed in Croatia with 137 patients having either a colorectal malignancy or other colorectal disease. Of these 137 patients, 53 were monitored postoperatively. There were 31 other patients that had no colonic disease and they served as the control group. The sensitivity was found to be 100% (all patients with precancerous and cancerous disorders had a positive test result) and the specificity was also an impressive 96.8% (30 of the 31 control patients had negative results i.e. no color change). The only patient of the controls that had a positive result was later found to have a sigmoid polyp, which would explain the positive test result in the initial screening; meaning that it was not really a 'false positive' reaction.

Of additional value, is that the test results continued to be positive in 60% (32 of 53) patients who were followed after their tumors were removed. This showed the persistence of the biochemical changes even though the cancers were already removed. Aside from providing evidence of the "field-effect" phenomenon of carcinogenic stimuli, on which the test is based on, the results also show its utility in monitoring patients for cancer recurrence as 5 of these 32 patients had a tumor reappearance within a year (*Anticancer Research* 21: 1247-1255, 2001)!

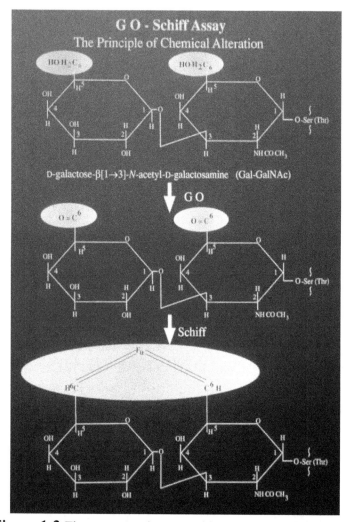

Figure 1-2 The enzyme galactose oxidase causes oxidation at C-6 positions of the carbohydrate marker galactose-*N*-acetyl-galacto-samine which then reacts with the Fuchsin dye of Schiff's reagent to yield a magenta color. The molecule in normal individuals or tissues is masked by sialic acid residues preventing such reaction by the enzyme.

METHOD OF PROCEDURE AND TYPICAL

RESULT

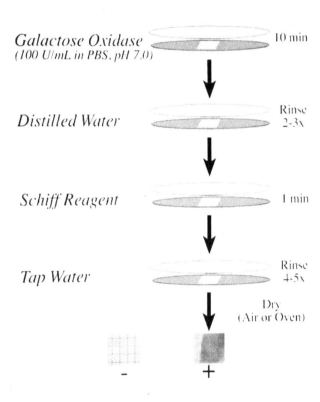

Figure 1-3 The steps in reaction are shown in this cartoon. Negative samples show no color whereas positive result is indicated by magenta coloration.

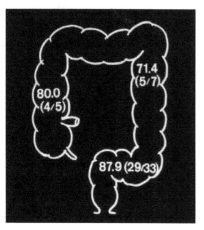

Figure 1-4: Schematic diagram of the human large intestine depicting the location of the cancers detected by the rectal mucus test. That the "field-effect" phenomenon is operational is proved by the detection of cancers in the various segments of the colon remote from the rectum where the mucus was sampled from. Note that 4 of 5 cancers (80%) of the ascending (or the right) colon, 5 of 7 (71.4%) of the descending (or the left) colon and 29 of 33 (87.9%) of the sigmoid colon were detected in the two studies by Dr. Sakamoto in Japan.

Lung Cancer Screening

"The study has indicated that T antigen [Gal-GalNAc] test of sputum is a sensitive method for the diagnosis of lung cancer. It may also be a promising approach for the massive screening of lung cancer in terms of its rapidity, economy and simplicity." X. Lai et al. 1995

That was in 1995. Unlike cancers of breast that have mammograms and that of colon the FOBT to screen for, when it comes to the cancer of the lungs there is not even a screening test in common use today, despite lung cancer being by far the deadliest of all the cancers. Only 10% of lung cancer patients survive more than 5 years if the disease is not caught in the early stages. And by the time the cancer shows up in the X-rays, it is simply too late...the one that robbed me of my dad and my favorite uncle.

As you have seen, the simple carbohydrate tumor marker D-galactose-β-[1→3]-N-acetyl-D-galactosamine (Gal-GalNAc) can be easily identified by a sequential galactose oxidase (GO)-Schiff reaction on rectal mucus samples from patients with colorectal cancer. Prior to detecting it in the rectal mucus samples, I had evaluated its feasibility by looking for it in the histological tissue sections first. Utilizing the concept of "field-effect" phenomenon operational in bringing the mucin changes in the large intestine, I had reasoned, why shouldn't the same principle be at work in other organs? If a rectal mucus sample can predict the presence or absence of a cancer in the colon, why not the sputum in lung cancer, nipple aspirate in breast cancer, prostatic massage secretion in prostate cancer and so on? So, I set out to study just that.

Gal-GalNAc is a Common Tumor Marker

In 1994 my student W. Mike Beasley and I had reported the results of our study on prostate cancer first. We tested the usefulness of the tumor marker Gal-GalNAc in differentiating the benign from the malignant and pre-malignant lesions of the prostate (as part of his dissertation towards a Masters' degree in Pathology). A sequential galactose oxidase technique (overnight incubation), followed by Schiff's reaction (15 minutes), was done on histological tissue sections of 65 carcinomas (cancers), 25 hyperplasias (benign lesions), 11 foci of adenosis, and 10 normal specimens. While none of the 35 benign prostates and 11 foci of adenosis expressed Gal-GalNAc (100% specificity), 62 (95.4% sensitivity) of 65 adenocarcinomas variably expressed the marker. We therefore proposed then that this simple technique may have potential use in routine histopathological analysis of prostatic specimens. That this marker, the technology and the principle could also serve as the basis of assays for early detection of prostatic malignancies by using prostatic massage secretion was also proposed (Shamsuddin & Beasley 1994).

Having determined that the principle is practicable in colon and prostate, I then set out to study other cancers. The expression of Gal-GalNAc determined in a total of 133 tissue samples from 81 cases of the carcinomas of the breast, ovary, pancreas, stomach, and endometrium and 52 cases of respective normal controls. None of the 52 cases of normal tissues (except 15 cases of stomach) showed expression of Gal-GalNAc. In contrast, 100% of adenocarcinomas from the breast (19 of 19), ovary (15 of 15), and pancreas (6 of 6), and 94.1% of stomach (16 of 17) cancers, and 91.7% (11 of 12) of uterine adenocarcinomas expressed Gal-GalNAc. The normal epithelia and their secretions in the vicinity of the carcinoma (within the "field") in the **breast, bronchus, endometrium, and pancreatic duct also expressed Gal-GalNAc in contrast to normal tissues** obtained from non-cancerous individuals, which were totally non-reactive. Thus, I had concluded that the tumor marker Gal-GalNAc recognized by Galactose Oxidase-Schiff sequence was highly expressed not only by a variety of adenocarcinomas but also by the apparently normal-appearing epithelia and their secretions in the vicinity of carcinomas. This confirmed my view about the operation of a field effect phenomenon by carcinogenic agent(s) in these organs as well, and set the stage for identification of the marker in these secretions for mass screening for these cancers too (Shamsuddin, A.M., *et al* 1995).

Chinese Study

That the principle of screening lung cancer by identifying Gal-GalNAc in sputum works for lung cancer has been first demonstrated by Dr. X Lai and colleagues at the Cancer Research Institute, China Medical University, Shenyang. They reported in the journal *Zhonghua Jie He He Hu Xi Za Zhi* in October 1995 (volume 18 No. 5: pages 285-286 [in Chinese] the results of their study on screening of sputum samples for early detection of lung cancer. Sputum specimens from 116 healthy persons and 216 cases of benign and malignant lung diseases were tested for the marker Gal-GalNAc using a strip test by galactose oxidase-Schiff sequence. The result showed that 165 of the 182 patients (90.7% sensitivity) with lung cancer, confirmed by cytology and histology, had positive results, whereas 22 of 116 (19.0%) healthy controls were positive (81.0% specificity). In 28 cases of patients whose cytology of sputa showed various degrees of dysplasia, 21 were found Gal-GalNAc positive, of which 15 patients were identified to have lung cancer in the follow-up study! In addition, three cases of early lung cancer in this study were also positive, suggesting that Gal-GalNAc is expressed at an earlier stage in the malignant process.

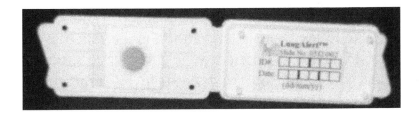

Figure 1-5: A sample LungAlert™ test strip showing positive reaction (magenta color) of the sputum of a lung cancer patient. The device consists of 2 leaves made of plastic which can be folded close; on the left-hand leaf is the special white paper on which the sputum sample is placed and reacted, the opposite leaf has identification data. The size is approximately 80% of the actual device (Courtesy of Dr. Michael Evelegh of PreMD, Inc., Toronto, Canada).

Canadian Study

It was not till 2001 when similar reports were presented by Drs. Miller and Cox from St. Joseph's Hospital/McMaster University, Hamilton, Ontario, Canada at the Annual Meetings of the American Thoracic Society and the American Association for Cancer Research. The test revealed 20 of 23 lung cancers among 76 patients. The other 53 patients were either healthy or had benign lung disease such as bronchitis. Even more germane to the issue of prevention is the fact that 13 of 15 cancers detected were early stage (Stage I and II out of four stages, Stage IV being most advanced).

*The front page of one of Canada's national newspapers-The National POST (Tuesday, May 22, 2001) quotes Dr. John Miller **"If these numbers pan out, this clearly is the best screening tool [for lung cancer] to come along in decades, or ever,"***

Breast Cancer Screening

As described earlier (reported in my 1995 *Cancer Research* paper), Gal-GalNAc is also expressed by the normal-looking breast tissue away from an obvious cancer by way of the field-effect pheno-

menon. Thus, the nipple aspirate from a breast har-
boring a cancer should express the marker. In a
pilot study published in the journal *Cancer* (volume 100, No. 12, pages 2549-2554, June 15, 2004),
Dr. Chagpar and colleagues from the M.D. Anderson Cancer Center in Houston Texas report the
potential utility of using nipple aspirate and Gal-
GalNAc in screening for breast cancer. They
investigated 23 women with biopsy confirmed,
unilateral stage I or II breast cancer. They took
samples (nipple aspirate by way of a suction cup
attached to a syringe) from both breasts prior to
surgery. Most, but not all of the women were able
to provide large enough fluid samples that could
then be evaluated (Figure 1-6). Since that was the

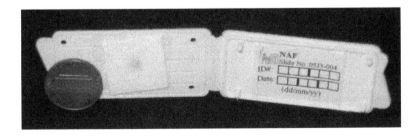

Figure 1-6: Positive nipple aspirate (magenta) on a sample
test strip. A US penny (1 cent coin) is included for size
comparison. Courtesy of Dr. Michael Evelegh of PreMD,
Inc., Toronto, Canada.

first clinical trial, for consistency prior to the actual test, it was determined what the minimum amount of fluid required for evaluation would be. It is quite possible that smaller samples may ultimately be useful. Based on the resulting color of the test strips, the investigators could tell which breast had a tumor. In other words, they could differentiate between a healthy and cancerous breast!

Once again, the theory is that cancer is the result of assault by carcinogenic stimuli; these carcinogens are in our environment such as in the air we breathe (tobacco smoke, asbestos or other air pollution), the food we eat [resulting in carcinogen attacking the stomach and the intestine etc. and also absorbed from the bowel and distributed by the blood to the colon as well as other organs], etc. Thus, it is most likely that the entire 'field' of exposed organ or tissue will be subjected to the carcinogenic insult; some cells being more susceptible than others will acquire unrepairable DNA damage and with repeated carcinogenic assaults and other promoting factors will progress to pre-cancer and cancer. The vast majority of the cells in this field however may not have the same fate, yet they would show telltale evidence of the assault by expressing the marker. In other words, expression of the marker is evidence of the cells' acquiring some damage and is shared by both cells that become cancerous and those who do not - "field-effect." The rectum is a part of the 'colorectal field' and a convenient sampling site. A cancer or polyp in the right (ascending), horizontal (transverse) or left (descending) colon is likely the result of such field exposure, but the rectal mucosal cells will most likely be expressing the same marker as the cancer far away. Likewise, the cancer in the lung could be anywhere but the mucosal cells which secrete mucus will be expressing the marker throughout much of the entire bronchial tree; thus, the coughed-up sputum is likely to be positive. And so on with the breast, the prostate, the pancreas etc.

How simple is the test? For lung cancer, all one has to do is cough-up the sputum, for breast cancer - give the nipple aspirate, for colon cancer – the rectal mucus sample following digital examination, and then reacting for less than 15 minutes in a 2-step process and look for magenta color.

CHAPTER 2

PREVENTION I

As you have gathered from the preceding, Gal-GalNAc technology and the principle of "field-effect" detect not only established cancer, but also cancers in very early stages including precancerous lesions and conditions; the latter carries a high risk of cancer at a subsequent time. Once a person is screened for cancer there are several possible outcomes: i) a malignancy is detected and patient has undergone appropriate therapy, b) an early-stage cancer is detected, c) the person is test negative therefore no further action may be necessary for him/her.

Not only are the individuals with a precancerous lesion and/or condition are at a high risk of cancer, those who have undergone treatment are also at an elevated risk for either a recurrence and/or a second (and occasionally a third) malignancy. These individuals need to be protected by prophylaxis. And then just because a person is screening test negative is no guarantee for being immune to cancer in the future; thus, it may be prudent for them to consider prevention as the incidence of many cancers increase with increasing age. This brings us to the topic of prevention by IP₆ & Inositol the main topic of the book:

IP₆ & Inositol

Almost every cell in our bodies contains a compound I consider to be one of nature's major contributors to good health – inositol. Inositol is counted among the members of the B-vitamin family. Particularly the nervous system, the brain, and the reproductive organs require a steady supply of this compound. In our fight against cancer, inositol plays a major role because it helps control cell growth. Our immune system is generally capable of keeping cancer cells in check, but cancer may spread if our immune functions become overwhelmed. Mounting body of research data from scientists around the world strongly suggests that inositol – and related substances called inositol phosphates – can prevent not just the formation, but also the spread of cancer.

From a chemical perspective, structurally inositol is similar to glucose and is thus considered a "sugar" (it does in fact have a sweet taste). Much more significant is however the fact that relatively modest changes to its chemical structure – for instance the addition of phosphate groups (which lead to the creation of a group called inositol phosphates or inositol polyphosphates - IPP) – can produce an array of biochemical effects. Inositol was originally named 'inos' (muscle in *Greek*) by Josef Scherer a German chemist, who more than 150 years ago, isolated the new molecule from muscle tissue. Inositol is a simple hexa-carbon carbohydrate derivative of glucose; to date nine inositol stereoisomers have been identified based on the position of OH groups on the ring; only four are physiologically active (please see Figure 2-1), and the most abundant in nature is *myo*-inositol.

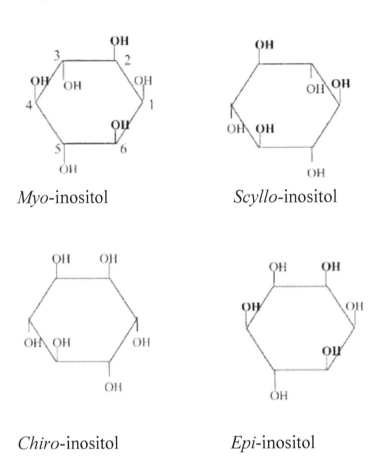

Myo-inositol

Scyllo-inositol

Chiro-inositol

Epi-inositol

Figure 2-1: Four of the stereoisomers of inositol; note the differences in the position of OH groups.

When all of the six carbons molecules in the ring are attached to phosphate groups, it is known as inositol hexaphosphate (IP₆, InsP₆). Figure 2-2 shows the chemical structure of inositol hexaphosphate.

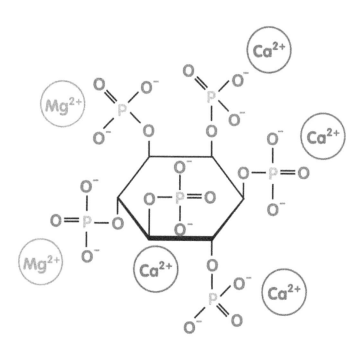

Figure 2-2: Chemical structure of calcium magnesium inositol hexaphosphate P = Phosphorus; O = oxygen.

The phosphate derivatives are named in accordance with the number of phosphate group attached to the inositol molecule. Given that there are six places on the inositol molecule where phosphates may attach, we can differentiate six forms of inositol phosphates:

1. Inositol monophosphate (IP_1);

2. Inositol bisphosphate (IP_2);

3. Inositol trisphosphate (IP_3)

4. And proceeding in this fashion all the way to IP_6, which is called inositol hexaphosphate, or inositol hexakisphosphate.

5. In recent days, inositols with 7 and 8 phosphates (IP_7, IP_8) known as inositol pyrophosphates have been discovered within our cells which also exert important biological functions.

Of particular importance for our cancer research is inositol hexaphosphate; though not the most precise, for convenience's sake I have adapted the abbreviation IP_6, which is also referred more accurately as $InsP_6$.

IP_6 was originally discovered in different plant seeds in 1855-1856 by T. Hartig, and was named "phytin" owing to its plant origin. In 1897 Winterstein named it inosite-phosphoric acid. Various molecular structures were proposed since then resulting in, as you can imagine some controversy till 1914 when Anderson presented it as *myo*-inositol-1,2,3,4,5,6, hexakis dihydrogen phosphate, a structure that has stood the test of time, till now that is. The process of its preparation was patented by Posternak (US Patent # 1,313,014 awarded to Ciba) in 1918 who named it phytic acid – a label that has stuck since then.

Chemically as you can see from the structure in Figure 2-2, IP_6 (inositol hexaphosphoric *acid*) can bind with cations such as Ca^{++}, Mg^{++}, Zn^{++}, Fe^{++} etc forming the salt – inositol hexaphosphate (a.k.a. phytate) which is how it exists in nature. The preceding also refers to chemical reactions in test-tubes whereby inositol hexaphosphoric *acid* binds with cations.

Beginning the early 1940's reports started to app-ear that certain populations who were consuming a high-IP_6-diet were deficient in Ca^{++}, Mg^{++}, Zn^{++}, Fe^{++}. Coupled with the fact that in the lab inositol hexaphosphoric *acid* binds with cations and named phytic *acid*, it became notorious as an "anti-nutrient." That inositol hexaphosphoric *acid* also has other chemical properties especially as an anti-oxidant with resultant industrial applications became evident. However, despite the recognition of it as an antioxidant, its great potential for human health benefits was largely ignored or remained unappreciated. Perhaps this was because the havoc oxidative damage causes were not known and the importance of antioxidants not realized until recently. In any event, crying "anti-nutrient" there have been a well-concerted effort in the agricultural sector to reduce or eliminate IP₆ from our diet by genetically engineering <u>l</u>ow <u>p</u>hytic <u>a</u>cid (lpa) mutants. It seems that some of the mutated crops and seeds acquire their own problems.

One hundred and thirty years following IP₆'s discovery, it was in 1987 that research in my laboratory has shown that this so-called anti-nutrient boosts immunity through natural killer cells and prevents and even shrinks cancers. We will discuss the issue of safety later. Suffice it to say here, that not only the "anti-nutrient" role has been disproven, but that IP₆ has also numerous health benefits are being appreciated.

To avoid any confusion, unless otherwise indicated, IP₆ in this book and elsewhere in my publications refers to the natural salt form: inositol hexa*phosphate*.

By removing the phosphate groups on IP₆ molecule it can revert back to inositol. Conversely, inositol may be converted to IP₆ by adding phosphate groups; the relationship is like the chicken and the egg. IP₆ and inositol are synergistic in their health effects. This means that the positive effects of IP₆ and inositol are enhanced when these substances are given in combination rather than individually. This has particular relevance for so-called "anticancer cocktails" where inositol is added to IP_6 in order to enhance the cocktail's effectiveness.

In experiments carried out in my laboratory, IP_6 has been shown to lead to a statistically significant reduction in certain types of cancers, such as those affecting the colon, the breast, the prostate, the liver, etc. These positive effects were shown to be both consistent and reproducible. Worldwide, scientists have been not only confirming, validating this research, but also are continually expanding on this vital work.

Throughout the book, I shall be referring to scientific studies done by various investigators including me, and I shall be referring to statistical significance and p-value. When is a study considered to be "statistically significant"? When it has generated results that all researchers accept as valid. For instance, a particular study may indicate that a specific treatment produces a positive effect; however, if the number of patients enrolled in the study (sample size) is insufficient, the study results may simply be due to chance. Scientific study protocol demands that the observations are proven to be not by chance. Thus, rigorous calculations are done to demonstrate whether or not the results are "statistically significant". Non-statistically significant results (i.e. chance observations) are therefore not readily acceptable neither by medical practitioners nor the scientific community at large, nor should it be accepted by the public. A *p*-value of 0.05 or less (<0.05) is considered significant, the lower the value (such as 0.01, 0.001 etc), the more the significance and the less it is likely to be a chance observation.

However, one must not totally ignore chance observations either, as historically they have led us to the discovery of new diseases and treatments; they break the ground for further large scale studies with large sample size and adequate controls to establish the disease or treatment. Most diseases including AIDS were initially detected as single or a cluster of few cases by some astute, keenly observant physician who followed-up on the observation(s) leading to larger studies and establishment of the disease. As an example, it was a single case observation by Dr. Alzheimer that established the eponymous disease we all are so painfully aware of now.

Facts about Inositol

Around the time of my initiating the anti-cancer experiments of IP_6 and inositol, biochemists have started to identify first IP_3 and later IP_4 initially in baker's yeasts, slime molds etc and more recently in mammalian cells. Though IP_6 have been known to occur in the plants, cereal grains and seeds since mid 1850's, and the existence of inositol within our body has been well known, my colleagues in IP_6 biochemistry research have not been investigating it until recently. Part of the reasons may be the difficulty in identification and lack of interdisciplinary research. We are only beginning to understand the essential roles various inositol compounds, especially inositol polyphosphates play in our bodies; we are at the beginning of our journey. Following are a few facts about inositol:

- Inositol is an essential compound (in this case, a nutrient) without which cells in artificial culture media cannot survive in a laboratory setting;

- Inositol has shown remarkable characteristics both in the prevention and the treatment of various cancers;

- Inositol has been used to treat psychiatric disorders;

- It has also shown positive effects in preventing the complications typically associated with diabetes mellitus;

- Recently it has been demonstrated that inositol itself is an antioxidant.

Facts about IP₆

Now, let me list just a few of the many established facts about IP₆:

1. That IP₆ (inositol hexaphosphoric *acid*) is an antioxidant has been known since the mid 1970's and it has found various industrial applicability. IP₆'s anti-oxidative properties imply that it can reverse the damaging effects caused by free radicals during oxidative processes within our bodies.

2. IP₆ also plays a role in the prevention of kidney stones;

3. IP₆ heightens the body's resistance to infections;

4. Furthermore, IP₆ serves to lower serum cholesterol and triglyceride levels – two of

the main risk factors in the development of heart disease;

5. IP$_6$ also prevents heart muscle damage during a heart attack;

6. IP$_6$'s positive effects extend even further, perhaps prolonging the life span of certain plant seeds. It is a well-known fact that certain seeds have the potential to remain viable for up to 400 years (i.e. they retain their ability to grow under suitable circumstances for an extended length of time). IP$_6$ may account for this considerable longevity.

7. Inositol phosphates play a key role in regulating the oxygen-carrying capacity of red blood cells; in fact, these compounds may be highly relevant in the treatment of sickle cell anemia.

There is no doubt in my mind that future research will continue to uncover more and more ways in which inositol derivatives benefit humans, animals, and plants. The examples cited above are just a few of many.

Among the inositol molecules, IP$_6$ has been my favorite subject of research. Claiming that IP$_6$ is "the aspirin of the 21st century" is perhaps even an understatement. IP$_6$'s potential is far greater than that of aspirin, not to mention that it is also much safe. Thus, my calling the combination of IP₆+ inositol as the Medicine for the Millennium is no hyperbole; it has already been here for one and one-half century, about 50 years more than aspirin and the number of health benefits we are discovering is only growing *without* the negative side-effects of most drugs, aspirin included! Others seem to agree.

> *"This new cancer-fighter derived from fiber may also prove to be a medicine for the new millennium." Jose Antonio, PhD, 1998*

In this book, I share research information about IP₆ & inositol - a gift nature gave us that we have yet to fully comprehend.

So, what is the source of inositol and IP₆? IP₆ and inositol are found abundantly in cereals and in legumes. You may be aware of the causality between diets high in fiber and the reduced incidence of certain types of cancer. This topic sets the stage for the subsequent chapters where I shall discuss the roles inositol and IP₆ play in the suppression of cancer and other disease, and how it all relates to the importance of dietary fiber.

CHAPTER 3

PREVENTION II

Mothers Know Best

Our mothers have always told us to eat healthy and we should have listened if we didn't! And they told us to eat a lot of fiber. The scientific community and the media finally caught up to the wisdom of our mothers. Over the past 50 years, fiber has received extensive press coverage. Unfortunately, people have been bombarded with a wide range of diverging opinions on the subject. Some of the headlines fiber has garnered include: "Fiber sweeps your intestines clean like a broom", "Oat bran rinses your body free of cholesterol", "Fiber fights cancer", "Fiber may fight cancer", "Fiber may not be as important in fighting cancer as previously believed", and so on, and so forth. The bottom line is, people were confused by numerous, sometimes pseudo-medical opinions and statements, yet rarely given the relevant facts.

What Should You Know About Fiber?

Our dietary fiber comes from the plants we eat. Dietary fiber is not truly digested in our bodies; neither our digestive enzymes nor the enzymes produced by our intestinal flora are able to fully decompose it. The flora that does some of the decomposition work consists of the multitudes of microorganisms that live harmlessly within our bodies - such as in the colon (but also on our skin). These bacteria provide essential and highly specific functions without which we would die. It has been estimated that we carry up to a kilogram of floral bacteria in our intestines alone.

Fiber can be classified according to its resistance to digestion:

- Insoluble fiber is highly resistant to digestion
- Soluble fiber is comparatively less resistant.

You may have heard that fiber is good for you because it increases the bulk of your stool. This is certainly the case and a good bulk density is essential for the normal elimination process. But the question arises, does *all* fiber perform this function, and to what extent?

As noted, fiber can be differentiated by the degree to which it resists digestion, and this has an impact on the size of the stool that is produced. In the intestines, soluble fiber is broken down to a greater extent than insoluble fiber; however, soluble fiber increases stool bulk only moderately whereas insoluble fiber, given its much higher water absorption capacity augments it to a greater extent.

Fiber's main components are the so-called polysaccharides – which is simply another name for carbohydrates. As you may remember from your chemistry lessons, carbohydrates consist of carbon, hydrogen, and of oxygen atoms. When these are rearranged in various configurations, different types of carbohydrates are created - among them cellulose, hemicellulose, pectins, gums, mucilages, and lignin.

In chemical terms, soluble fiber (consisting of pectins, gums, mucilages, and some hemicellulose molecules) can be partly digested in our intestines. In contrast, insoluble fiber is not degraded well in our gut. Among the insoluble fiber constituents we include lignin, cellulose, as well as some hemicellulose molecules. Given a choice of selecting the type of fiber that will best bulk up your stool, insoluble fiber is the material of choice.

What kinds of foods should we eat to get soluble and insoluble fiber? Soluble fiber is found in fruits and vegetables, and in some grains (in oats, for instance). Cereals, notably whole-grain cereals represent the major source of insoluble fiber. Fruits and vegetables also contain some insoluble fiber. The richest source of insoluble fiber is the outer coating (the broken husks) of cereal grains – also known as bran.

When we eat foods that are rich in fiber, we typically consume them in different forms. Firstly, we may ingest fiber while eating whole foods: unprocessed ("whole") cereal grains, beans and peas (legumes), fruits, and vegetables. Secondly, we may eat processed foods that are rich in fiber – such as wheat bran, corn bran, and bran from rice. We may also ingest fiber that has been isolated and purified – this would consist of cellulose, pectins, gums, and lignin components. A third way we sometimes eat fiber is when we take it for specific (medical) reasons. A good example is a certain species of plantain (with the botanical name *Plantago ovata).* The husks of this plantain's seeds are used as a laxative because they have strong hydrophilic (i.e., water absorbing) properties. The seeds of another plantain (*Plantago psyllium)* – called psyllium seeds – are also used for the same purpose.

The benefits of fiber for good health have long been recognized. Much of the initial research was conducted by Dr. George Oettle of South Africa. The credit for having advocated the benefits of dietary fiber and its role in preventing colon cancer is generally given to Dr. Dennis Burkett. Dr. Burkett wrote about fiber's health benefits in a

1969 article in the journal *Lancet.* However, it must be recognized that a researcher from India – Dr S.L. Malhotra – published information on the connection between fiber and colon cancer in 1967 – thus preceding Dr Burkett's work by at least a year.

In India, eating habits vary greatly from region to region; there are also differences between the various religious groups. Dr. Malhotra conducted an extensive study of these dietary habits, comparing the foods eaten in India's North with those eaten in the South. He was a pioneer in demonstrating in a conclusive manner that people who eat a diet high in fiber have a lower risk of developing certain diseases, among them colon cancer. He made the observation that colon cancer was significantly less prevalent in Northern India than in the South. He noted that "While the North Indian diets are rich in roughage, cellulose, and vegetable fibers, these are almost completely lacking in the South Indian diets."

The question arises how fiber is able to inhibit colon cancer. At least two reasons can be given. Firstly, fiber can indeed act like a broom that sweeps out our intestines. It does so by absorbing (i.e., sticking to) cancer-causing or cancer-promoting chemicals in the gut (these are known as carcinogens). The presence of fiber can also speed up our stool's transit time. One of the benefits associated with our stool exiting more quickly is that cancer-promoting or cancer-causing chemicals have less time to interact with the cells in our intestines.

A failure to neglect our "housekeeping duties" can lead to the development of health problems such as diverticulitis – an inflammatory condition quite prevalent in middle age where the diverticulii - small sacs or pouches found in the wall of the colon – become plugged with stagnant stool. Diverticulosis refers to a condition where a number of such pockets develops and then become inflamed (diverticulitis). This can lead to painful discomfort; in rare cases, also to obstructions in the colon, perforations, even bleeding.

Even though Dr. Malhotra was the first to present and publish scientific evidence of fiber's health benefits, it was Dr. Burkett who popularized the concept, as he published and lectured widely on the topic. His lectures often included slides that demonstrated vividly how fiber benefits our intestines. As a consequence; a high fiber diet remained a popular notion for some 30 years. Today, unfortunately, it appears that the scientific community, the government, and private agencies (through their research grants) have quietly abandoned further research on fiber. Why?

The reasons for this are not entirely clear to me. One possible explanation is that fiber, as you now know, is a rather complex substance that contains many different nutrients. To illustrate, let's look at rice bran. It contains protein, healthy oil, vitamins (for instance vitamin E), antioxidants (for example γ-oryzanol), lecithin, as well as inositol and its family of phosphate-containing molecules. During the metabolic processes in our bodies, many carbohydrates such as inositol end up containing phosphorus, the atom found in phosphate groups. If we now compare rice bran to other types of brans, we will find that other brans may contain some of the same nutrients found in rice bran; however, they may also include other, different components. You can see that any attempts to establish which substance performs which function in the body becomes quite a challenge!

A further reason why interest in fiber has waned is to be found in the surging interest in competing research that looks at the risks associated with a diet high in fat. More and more studies attempt to correlate a high fat intake with the risks of developing breast cancer, as well as other cancers. It appears that investigating these facts became more popular than carrying out further research on fiber.

But if you think about it for a moment, one aspect that is perhaps neglected is the fact that when one eats a diet high in fat and protein, one's fiber intake is automatically reduced. Steak and eggs, bacon, and sausage may appeal more than a bowl of salad or beans. Your personal experience may indicate that while you're having a filet mignon, you are likely to cut down on foods like bread, salad, and side vegetables. But by reducing the amount of fiber we eat while increasing our intake of fat and protein comes at the expense of something very valuable to our health: The benefits that have been clearly shown to be associated with fiber.

In conclusion, we may perhaps find that it is specifically the reduction of our fiber intake – rather than an increase in fat consumption – that contributes most strongly to the potential development of colon cancer.

Not All Fibers are Same

During the cell division process, a replication of our genetic material (the DNA) takes place. It is at this time that our genes (which are found in our cells' nuclei) literally unravel. Our genes are made up of DNA double strands. These now uncoil because the body requires them to be open so that each DNA strand may be copied for the production of a new "daughter" cell. During the DNA copying process – where our genetic material has an open structure – our DNA is particularly susceptible to attacks by cancer-causing agents. The longer the cell division process is extended, the higher the risk of such attacks. In addition, during each copying process, there is also the risk of inaccurate copying.

If for some reason the number of cell divisions is increased beyond what is typical, there is a two-fold risk that mutations will occur, and that the DNA could be damaged during the copying process. It is a characteristic of cancer that it is associated with an increase in the rate of cell divisions that keep on going in an uncontrolled manner; in fact, increased cell division is a first step in getting cancer. Scientists make use of this phenomenon when they study cancers in the laboratory. They expose cells or animals to certain agents that have been shown to increase the rate of cell division. In doing so, they increase the incidence of experimental cancers.

As discussed above, researching the health effects of fiber is a complicated endeavor. To further compound this complexity, it is known that the effects fiber produces can vary greatly based on a number of dietary factors.

Interestingly, lab tests with rodents have shown that certain diets high in fiber may actually *increase* the rate of cell division in the colon. Dr. R. Lucien Jacobs has demonstrated that corn and oat bran can increase the incidence of experimentally-induced colon cancers in rats. Dr. Jacobs explained that the colon's level of acidity was bolstered by a diet high in oat and in corn fibers. Specifically, as the flora breaks these types of fiber down in the bowel, fatty acids are produced. The cells that line our intestines then use these fatty acids as fuel. The problem is that the energy derived from this fuel has been shown to increase both cell division and cell proliferation. In these experiments, 20% of the rats' diet consisted of oat bran – a very high percentage. To compensate for the comparative lack of calories found in this high-fiber diet, the rats increased their food intake (the higher amount of food they ate may be a further factor affecting their health).

Other studies have shown a significant increase in colon tumors when there was a high level of bran in the diet (i.e., 20%). In contrast, when rats were given a diet that contained significantly lower levels of corn bran (of only 4.5%), the number of tumors was reduced.

Next, let us look at different kinds of brans to see how they factor into the equation. When rats were fed rice and soybean bran – even at the 20% level, and even when their diet was high in fat - no significant influence on the number of tumors was detected. Even though it may be difficult to compare such results directly with other studies, given the variations in the amounts of fiber and of fat – such experimental studies indicate that the type of fiber that is ingested plays a significant role.

Now, let's turn our attention to largescale studies of human populations, researching how fiber relates to the incidence and distribution of cancers. Several groups of researchers have undertaken this kind of work. They have investigated the relationships between fiber and various diseases, and more specifically looked at the connections between the type of fiber we eat and its role in the development of cancer.

Among these researchers is Dr. David G. Zaridze, who discussed these complex interactions in a 1983 article that appeared in the *Journal of the National Cancer Institute*. Dr. Zaridze believes that dietary factors are a key risk factor for the development of cancer, certainly ranking at least second in importance (right after tobacco). He considers the correlation between diet and cancers to be most direct for large bowel cancer.

The bottom line is that not all high fiber diets correlate directly and positively with a lower incidence of cancer (for instance with colon cancer). Only high fiber diets based specifically on cereals – notably diets that include rice and wheat – have been shown to be strongly and consistently linked to a lower frequency of colon cancer. What exactly do cereals contain that makes them unique and distinct from other diets also high in fiber?

How Does Fiber Prevent Cancer?

The outer bran layers of cereals and legumes (which include beans and peas) consist largely of soluble fiber. Contained within these bran layers is the important "sugar" we discussed earlier – inositol hexaphosphate (IP$_6$) – you may recall previously called phytate; it has also been loosely called phytic acid. It is important to keep in mind that phytic acid is inositol hexaphosphoric *acid*, where as phytate is a salt form, such as calcium-magnesium inositol hexaphosphate.

"One component of insoluble fiber, phytic acid [IP$_6$], has been proven to be particularly effective in preventing colon cancer induction in models." John H. Weisburger et al (1993).

In this context, please do not misunderstand the term "acid". Calling IP$_6$ "phytic acid" may give the erroneous impression that it refers to a corrosive substance similar perhaps to sulfuric acid or nitric acid. This is not the case - the term "acid" simply refers to a compound's chemical structure, making no reference at all to its degree of "acidity". In fact, there are numerous acids that are highly beneficial for one's health: Two that come immediately to mind are folic acid a B-vitamin and ascorbic acid (vitamin C). Inositol hexaphosphoric *acid* however does not exist in nature. Thus, henceforth, throughout the book I shall refer to IP₆ as the salt form which occurs in nature as Calcium-Magnesium-IP₆ or those specifically prepared for experimental purposes such as Sodium-IP₆, Potassium-IP₆ etc.

Where do we find IP₆?

IP₆ is a natural component found in nuts, legumes, most cereals; sesame and corn contains the highest amount – about 5-6%; rice bran may contain as high as up to 8.7%.

In the *World Review of Nutrition and Diet* (1987), Drs. Barbara Harland and Donald Oberleas reported that mature soybean seeds contain as much as 2.58% of IP₆ (in contrast to various soy-based compounds, which contain much smaller amounts). Where *exactly* in seeds does the IP₆ reside? It depends on the type of seed.

Table 3-1: IP₆ Content of Various Seeds

Food	IP₆ Content (in percent)
Corn	0 – 6.4
Wheat	1.1 - 4.8
Sesame	5.3
Beans	2.5
Rice	2.2
Peanuts	1.9
Sunflower	1.9
Soybeans	0.1 – 1.8
Soybean concentrate (textured)	1.5
Barley	1.0
Peas	0.9
Oats	0.8

- In monocotyledons (flowering plants whose seed embryos contain a *single* seed leaf or cotyledon), IP₆ is stored inside the particles that make up the bran layer (the aleuronic layer). Two examples are rice and wheat;

- In contrast, in dicotyledons (flowering plants that have *two* embryonic seed leaves or cotyledons), IP₆ is stored within the seed as a salt of calcium and magnesium (aka phytin). Castor, peanut, cotton, and beans are prominent examples of dicotyledon seeds that contain IP_6.

For cereals, such as rice, wheat, and rye, today's standard *milling procedures lead to removal of the bran* (the seeds' outer layer). Because it is precisely here that IP_6 is heavily concentrated such processing invariably reduces the total amount of IP_6 left in these seeds. White (or polished) rice may serve as an example of this unfortunate processing fad of recent decades – it makes this food deficient in IP_6 (recall that rice contains up to 2.2% IP_6 whereas rice bran contains up to 8.7%!). Corn is also an interesting example. It is unique in that most of its IP_6 (roughly 88%) is found in a concentrated form within the germ portion of the kernel. If corn is "de-germed", it may also become IP_6 deficient. Table 3-2 shows the IP_6 of various breads.

Table 3-2: Bread IP₆ Content

Type of Bread	IP₆ Content (in percent)
Corn	1.36
Whole wheat	0.56
Rye	0.41
Pumpernickel	0.16
Raisin	0.09
French	0.03
White	0.03

But where do the seeds get their IP_6 from? Simple; the soil! While the isomer of IP_6 in the seeds is *myo-* form that found in the soil is of *scyllo-* form. Thus, from the soil through the seeds and plant stems it goes to the grains and by eating cereal grains we consume it. Does it get absorbed from our gut or does it become degraded? For long it has been assumed that IP_6 cannot be absorbed from the gut, be it in humans or other species. But that has changed!

Where is the Fiber – IP₆ Connection?

The 1985 edition of the journal *Cancer* contains an editorial written by Dr. Ernst Graf and his associate John Eaton. The two researchers (who were working at the Pillsbury Company at the time) were curious whether it was fiber or IP_6 that provided the actual health benefits. In the editorial, Drs. Graf and Eaton reviewed a study on the health effects of fiber which compared the eating habits of people in Finland with those in Denmark. It was found that the Finnish population thrives on a diet rich in cereals and that it thereby consumed a lot of IP_6. In contrast, the Danes had a total fiber intake double that of the Finns, yet their diet contained less IP_6. Perhaps surprisingly, it had been known that the incidence of colon cancer among the Finns was only half as great as it was among the Danes. In other words, even though the Danes reportedly ate twofold the amount of fiber, they ended up having twice as much cancer! How can this phenomenon be explained? Drs. Graf and Eaton suggest that IP_6 is the key. They surmised that it is the high amounts of phytate (IP_6) in the Finnish diet that contributed to the observed health benefits owing to its antioxidant property.

A high consumption of corn and of dried beans is the most prominent characteristic of the typical diet among rural South African Blacks. People most commonly eat a type of porridge prepared from the boiling of corn that was pounded at home, or they use coarsely ground corn to prepare this dish. The average South African Black consumes about 680 g of corn per day. Since corn contains up to 6% IP_6, the average person thus ingests up to about 40.8 g of IP_6 per day [how much of that is actually absorbed is however not clear]. As per the observations made in 1970 (and published in 1980) by Dr. Monte Modlin of the Medical School of Cape Town, at that time 4.5 million Whites lived in urban areas together with 5.1 million blacks. Based on this population distribution, the astonishing result surfaced that over a nine-year time span (between 1971 and 1979), one in 510 White patients was admitted to the school's main teaching hospital with kidney stones, but - in stark contrast - only one in 44,298 Blacks was there for the same reason! What possible explanation could account for the vastly lower incidence of kidney stones (and of other diseases) in urban blacks compared to urban whites? It appears that in spite of having altered their eating habits to a certain extent (i.e., consuming more meat), urban blacks nonetheless continued to eat corn as part of their traditional diet – and this may in fact have contributed to their much lower incidence of kidney stone.

These are only two examples of the beneficial actions of healthy diet *via* IP₆ in preventing many of our ailments.

CHAPTER 4

ABOUT IP$_6$

So Why Not Eat A Lot Of Fiber?

From the preceding, it would be a natural question to ask: Since high fiber diets such as cereals and legumes are rich in IP$_6$ and Inositol, can we get the same benefit by eating them? The answer is Yes and No!

Yes, we must eat a healthy diet rich in wholegrain cereals and legumes to stay healthy and reduce the chances of diseases due to unhealthy dietary habits. Unfortunately during the past half a century or more, it appears that the types of cereal grain we are eating have changed. Most serious is the trend of polishing them for an attractive look. But as I mentioned before, polishing rice or wheat results in loss of the very important nutrients, including IP₆ and inositol. Thus, though attractive it may be to some, polished grains are detrimental to the health of all of us. Indeed, Dr. Chatenoud and colleagues from Milan, Italy have reported in the *International Journal of Cancer* (vol 77: pages 24-28, 1998) the relationship between the frequency of consumption of whole grain food and the risk of selected neoplasms (tumors, both benign and malignant) using data from an integrated series of case-control studies conducted in northern Italy between 1983 and 1996. The study included 181 histologically confirmed neoplasms (tumors) of the oral cavity and pharynx, 316 from esophagus, 745 from stomach, 828 from colon, 498 from rectum, 428 from liver, 60 from gallbladder, 362 from pancreas, 242 from larynx, 3,412 from breast, 750 from endometrium, 971 from ovary, 127 from prostate, 431 from bladder, 190 from kidney, 208 from thyroid 208; and 80 Hodgkin's disease, 200 non-Hodgkin's lymphomas, and 120 cases of multiple myeloma. Controls were 7,990 patients admitted to hospital for acute, non-neoplastic conditions, unrelated to long-term modifications in diet and not likely to have been caused by tobacco or alcohol use. The authors conclude:

"High intake of whole grain foods consistently reduced risk of neoplasm at all sites, except thyroid...even in the absence of a unequivocal and satisfactory biological interpretation, the consistency of the patterns observed indicate that, in this population, higher frequency of whole grain food intake is an indicator of reduced risk of several neoplasms." Chatenoud et al 1998.

And cancer is not the only scourge that is related to our dietary habit, particularly related to high-fiber diet. Drs. Curhan, Willett, Knight and Stampfer from Brigham and Women's Hospital in Boston prospectively examined, during an 8-year period, the association between dietary factors and the risk of incident symptomatic kidney stones among 96,245 female participants in the Nurses' Health Study II. They documented 1,223 incident symptomatic kidney stones during 685,973 person-years of follow-up.

"Phytate [IP₆] intake was associated with a reduced risk of stone formation...dietary phytate [IP6] may be a new, important, and safe addition to our options for stone prevention." Curhan et

al Archives of Internal Medicine vol 164, pages 885-891, April 26, 2004.

Thus, these epidemiological studies demonstrate that eating a healthy diet rich in fibers, particularly cereals and legumes is the way to go. But, we must also keep in mind that we are being increasingly assaulted by all the noxious substances that are polluting our environment, many of which are also cancer-causing agents or carcinogens. Thus, there is a need not only to eat healthy, but also to ensure added protection. And here is the explanation for the answer "*No*" – the amounts of IP₆ as you have seen in Tables 3-1 and 3-2 are variable depending on the sources. One must eat a huge amount of those food items to get enough IP₆ and Inositol, particularly for added protection of those at a high risk for various diseases; hence the supplement. You do not have to take my word for it; experimental studies done in my lab on breast cancer models and by Drs. Ohkawa & Ebisuno and their colleagues in Japan on kidney stone illustrate that as well (later in this chapter).

Lessons Learnt From Experimental Models of Breast Cancer

Today, we know that IP$_6$ fights cancer more effectively than high fiber. In order to develop an understanding of why this is the case, I would like to review an experiment that was specifically designed to establish which nutrient was most effective in slowing down mammary (i.e. breast) cancer in rats.

A great majority of the studies undertaken to investigate the links between diet and breast cancer focused on the role fat plays; in contrast, only a handful ever studied the effects of fiber. Research studies conducted in the lab as well as population studies indicate that a diet high in fat and calories yet low in fiber - typical and prevalent in the Western world heighten the risk for developing breast cancer.

The data that has come out of such studies has however been difficult to interpret. One reason for this is that diets high in fat are typically also low in fiber and that consequently, it has not been clearly established whether an increase in the occurrence of cancer should be:

1. Associated with the negative impacts of fat;

2. Attributed to a lack of fiber in the diet;

3. Or both.

There is an exception to every rule, and in this case, we have come across an interesting deviation - the typical Finnish diet which is both high in fiber and in fat. Perhaps unexpectedly, study results reported by Dr. D.P. Rose in 1992 and by Dr. H. Adlercreutz and colleagues in 1994, seem to indicate that the mortality from breast cancer (i.e. its death rate) is markedly lower in Finland than in the United States. Why?

In 1994, Dr. Zang and colleagues conducted a study among Hispanic, Black, and Caucasian college students in New York City. The purpose of the study was to determine whether there were any diet-related factors that could explain the dissimilar rates of breast cancer among these study groups. The study concluded that the Caucasian students were most susceptible to developing breast cancers compared to their Black and Hispanic classmates. At least in part, the Caucasians' higher risk was explained by dietary differences among the various groups of students. It was noted that both the Hispanic and the Black students consumed larger amounts of protective substances (directly as part of their regular diets). It is believed that the Hispanic students received such beneficial ingredients primarily from beans while the black students got them from fruits and vegetables. In contrast, the diets of the White students enrolled in the study were found to be more deficient in these substances.

A number of additional studies also point to the great impact our diet has, showing that dietary factors excluding fat, can affect the risk of developing breast cancer. Among these studies, I mention experiments carried out by Dr. de Stefanie and his colleagues in 1997, by Dr. Dunn in 1994, and by Drs. Cleaver and Smith in 1995.

Because it was already known that eating wholegrain cereals can reduce the risk of developing certain intestinal diseases (including colon cancer and appendicitis), we decided to study whether these cereals would also show a positive effect on breast cancer. It had already been established that IP₆ was found abundantly in the bran of certain mature seeds - for example in wheat. Furthermore, previous studies had also indicated that IP₆ in its pure form (i.e. without the bran) was a very powerful anticancer agent. So potent in fact that it could prevent cancer in very early stages - even while it was still undetectable. Before I delve into related studies in more detail, it is imperative that you first become acquainted with some of the terminology used to describe cancer during its various stages of formation.

Cancers Develop In Stages

The etymology of the term "cancer" can likely be traced back to the Latin word for "crab". This is a fitting analogy because cancer literally "adheres to any part that it seizes upon in an obstinate manner like the crab".

It is vital that you understand that cancer does not just appear overnight – out of the blue, so to speak. In order for cancer to develop, a whole series of complex interactions involving genetic, hereditary, and environmental factors must come into play. For instance, harmful environmental influences might include an exposure to toxic substances, such as chemicals, radiation from the sun or, from anthropogenic (i.e. caused by human) activity (x-rays), and even viruses. Furthermore, we know that diet plays a crucial role - it can greatly influ-

ence the actual outcome that may result from interplay of the various contributing factors.

Before a cancer can establish itself and ultimately
overpower the body's immune system, an entire
sequence of steps must occur. In situations where
a cancer is triggered by an exposure to a chemical
substance (either as an event deliberately set in
motion in the lab; or the result of an unintended
environmental exposure), we can distinguish two
main phases:

1. Stage one: A cancer is initiated;
2. Stage two: The cancer is promoted.

In our specific example, a certain chemical acts as
the initiator - it induces changes in our cells that
heighten the likelihood they will become cancerous. The process of cancer initiation by itself however does not produce cancer. A specific chemical
may indeed cause lasting damage to a cell's DNA
(i.e. to its genetic material), but a so-called promoter is then necessary in order to turn that damaged
cell into one that is cancerous. A cancer promoter
might:

- Consist of another chemical;

- Be a source of radiation (such as x-rays or UV rays from sun exposure);

- It could also be a virus.

Just as a cancer initiator cannot cause the disease on its own, the same principle applies to the promoter – by itself, it will not cause cancer. It is only when an initiator works in conjunction with a promoter that a cancer can be produced. This statement is however mitigated by the fact that a promoter does not have to be present immediately following a cancer initiation. In fact, a cancer-promoting factor may appear much, much later, thus explaining why some cancers take years to develop. A prominent example of this is asbestos, which as you might know can lead to lung cancer. Asbestos is the cancer initiator. As we have seen above, a cancer promoter is also required for the formation of lung cancer; in this case, smoking can act as the promoter. In my dad's case, he developed his lung cancer 20+ years after he stopped smoking!

It is well known that even when a person has been exposed to an initiator and is subsequently also exposed to a promoter, cancer will not necessarily result in every instance. This auspicious fact can be explained by the strength (health) of one's immune system. Tough, healthy immune defenses have the capacity to allow the body to repair its own damaged DNA (at least to a certain extent).

Our bodies have the power to produce enzymes that can cut and remove damaged (broken) DNA, thus enabling damaged cells to heal. However, our ability to produce such enzymes hinges to a significant degree on the quality of our diet. Our diet must provide the necessary raw materials. Enzymes, which are formed from proteins – require the presence of vitamins and minerals as so-called cofactors. If these are missing, an enzyme cannot function properly. Repair of double-strand breaks in DNA is essential for maintaining the stability of the genome, failure to repair may result in loss of genetic information, chromosomal translocation, and even cell death. Two mechanisms for this repair has been described – homologous recombination or non-homologous end-joining, you may be interested to know that IP₆ has been demonstrated to stimulate non-homologous end-joining; it has been proposed to be brought about by the binding of IP₆ to the DNA-dependent protein kinase DNA-PK$_{cs}$.

Now that you have some familiarity with the processes that potentially create cancer, let's review some studies specifically designed to find ways to stop cancer.

In my lab, a study with rats was carried out to investigate to what extent a diet high in fiber (bran) and rich in IP_6 would show a "dose-response inhibition" toward mammary cancer. What do we mean by dose-response inhibition? The term means that a known dose of a specific test substance (in this instance, bran or IP_6) will correspond to a measurable degree of cancer suppression. Typically, the more of a test substance one "applies", the greater the degree of cancer inhibition – all within reason, of course.

In our specific study, we fed rats with a diet high in fiber - at three levels consisting of 5%, 10%, and 20% of bran, respectively. The diet was started two weeks prior to the administration of a carcinogen – in this case, a substance called 7,12-dimethyl-benz[a] anthracene (DMBA). The goal of the experiment was to ascertain whether a cereal bran rich in IP_6 would exert the same protective effect as pure IP_6 administered on its own. To validate the experiment, a control group of animals was fed with a control diet, which consisted of the same food the other rats received, except the bran. The control group was however given IP_6 in their drinking water. The amount of IP_6 added to the water equaled the quantity of IP_6 given to the group of rats that received the most bran. 0.4% IP_6 was added to the drinking water, an amount that corresponds approximately to the IP_6 content found in the 20% bran diet. In human terms, this amount of IP_6 in the water would roughly equal to 500 mg to 1000 mg of IP_6 - if taken in a capsule form by a 70 kg person.

After the carcinogen has been administered, the rats were put on these diets for a full 29 weeks. At this time-point we discovered that:

- The rats fed with a 5% bran diet had a 16.7% reduction in the incidence of tumors;

- The rats receiving a diet consisting of 10% bran showed a reduction in tumor incidence of 14.6%;

- Finally, the rats that had received the 20% bran diet were found to have an 11.4% lower incidence of tumors.

However, when we analyzed these data statistically, these findings are not significant. Statistical tests told us that there is not enough of a difference between the rats that received bran in their diet and those that received none. In order to be considered statistically significant (p value equal to or less than 0.05), the results achieved would have to be confirmed by specific statistical formulas standard in scientific studies. Nevertheless, here are some further interesting results from this study:

The rats that received a dose of 0.4% IP₆ in their drinking water (which corresponds to the amount of IP₆ found in the 20% bran diet), showed a reduction in the incidence of tumors by 33.5%; in addition, there were 48.8% fewer tumors per animal. Here, the difference *is* statistically significant.

In summary, the study revealed that feeding the rats with additional dietary fiber (in the form of bran) resulted in only a very modest inhibitory effect which was not statistically significant. And, we did not see a dose-dependent response; feeding the animals with more bran did not result in a heightened cancer-suppressing effect.

Now, let's look at the rats that were given IP_6 in their drinking water (as stated, this occurred in doses equivalent to about 500 mg to 1000 mg for 70 kg humans). Here, the results do show a statistically significant reduction in the number of tumors, their incidence, and multiplicity (i.e. the number of tumors per animal). In the control group of animals (which received no IP_6 and no bran), the number of "palpable" tumors – defined as tumors that can be identified by means of touch – amounted to 73. The number of palpable tumors in the IP_6 group was however only 31. In those animals that had received pure IP_6 in their drinking water, we saw a statistically significant reduction (of 57.2%) in tumors.

Another key finding of the study was that pure IP_6 greatly reduced the extent to which tumors multiplied. Compared to the group treated with IP_6, we found more tumors per animal among those rats that had received the carcinogen alone, or among those that had received an exclusive fiber diet.

While tumors were still seen in those animals subjected to DMBA but given pure IP_6, it is noteworthy that 90% of these rats had only one or two tumors. In the group of animals that received only

DMBA, 45% of the rats produced three or more tumors (please refer to Table 4-1). In the group of animals receiving bran, between 25% and 42% of the rats had three or more tumors. These results indicate that only IP$_6$ administered in a pure form reduces the number of tumors per animal.

Four control animals not subjected to a treatment with carcinogens (and not given any bran or IP$_6$), still developed some palpable tumors; the tumors they produced were however non-cancerous (or benign – fibroadenomas). Spontaneously appearing tumors (those that appear in rats even without being exposed to carcinogens) were also discovered in 20% of the animals given the high fiber diet; however, no such tumors were found in the IP$_6$ group. It thus appears that IP$_6$ had a protective effect, preventing the development of spontaneously appearing mammary tumors.

In comparison to the animals subjected to the carcinogen DMBA, the rats receiving 0.4% IP$_6$ in their drinking water were the only animals to show a statistically significant reduction of tumor incidence.

Table 4-1: Comparison of the effects of bran v pure IP_6 in suppression of mammary cancer

Treatment / Diet Group	Tumor Incidence	Tumors per Rat	Rats with ≥ 3 Tumors
DMBA	79.0%	2.8	47%
DMBA + 20% bran	70.0%	3.1	36%
DMBA + 04% IP_6	52.6%	2.2	15%

DMBA = 7,12-dimethyl-benz[a] anthracene. Source: Adapted from Vucenik, Yang, and Shamsuddin (1997).

The decrease in the percentage of rats showing three or more tumors per animal was statistically significant. It is further noteworthy that those rats that received the 20% bran diet did not show a reduction in the incidence of cancer – even though they had been fed the same amount of IP_6 (i.e., 0.4%) as the animals receiving pure IP_6.

Taking IP_6 in a pure form may thus be a far more suitable approach to cancer prevention than forcing oneself to gulp down copious amounts of fiber. An article in the *Washington Post* dated March 14,

1989 – which reported on some of my research previously published in the cancer journal *Carcinogenesis* - came to a similar conclusion. *Post* reporter Larry Thompson concluded:

> *"[T]he American population may not have the gorge itself on fiber to prevent cancer after all."*

Having established that taking pure IP₆ seems far more reasonable and effective than getting it *via* bran, the question arises *why is this case?* There is a simple answer to this question.

The IP₆ found in whole fiber, bran, or in cereals is bound to proteins. For IP₆ to fight cancer effectively, it must reach the areas affected by a cancer or other disease. To get there, IP₆ must first be absorbed from the gut; it must then be transported in the bloodstream. For this to occur, IP₆ must initially be freed from the protein and other complexes to which it is bound. So, it's a long process during which period the enzymes, especially the phosphatases (those who chop off the phosphate groups, in this case from IP₆) have ample time to degrade IP₆.

Studies on Kidney Stone Prevention

Similar results have been demonstrated in prevention of kidney stone. Drs. Ohkawa and Ebisuno and their colleagues have reported back in December of 1984 that the urinary calcium excretion and its absorption in the intestine were reduced significantly by rice bran or phytin in rats fed high calcium diets, while there were no significant decreases with a low calcium diet. In a clinical study, 70 patients with idiopathic hypercalciuria was treated with rice bran (10 g twice daily) for 1 month to 3 years. Rice bran caused a significant decrease in urinary calcium excretion in most, if not all the treated patients. Evidence of stones had decreased clearly among patients treated with rice bran for 1 to 3 years. The authors attribute the results to IP$_6$. And here is the point: Eating 10 gm of rice bran twice daily may not be particularly appealing when one can get the same effect by taking much smaller amount of IP$_6$ supplement.

As alluded to earlier, in our intestines, of the various enzymes, the ones that are germane to our discussion are phosphatases; those that remove phosphates from IP$_6$ are called phytase (also found in food) since they break down 'phytate' thereby rendering IP_6 powerless in the fight against cancer. It has been shown that the longer it takes for the IP_6 to be released from the whole fiber; the more it potentially becomes degraded by this enzyme. Therefore, even though a diet high in fiber may have a lot of IP_6, you may never enjoy its full impact. That is why I consider pure IP_6 to be a much better solution – the body is able to absorb it fully before phytase can destroy it, as it is rather quickly absorbed.

What about possible side effects?

In our experiment, we also recorded each animal's weight (all of the rats received an identical amount of calories with their food). We found that neither the addition of bran to the diet, nor the addition of IP_6 to the drinking water had any negative effects in this respect – body weights remained very similar across all test groups. Since some researchers have voiced concerns that a chronic administration of fiber or IP_6 might lead to mineral deficiencies, we measured each animal's blood serum levels of calcium, magnesium, zinc, and iron. Neither the fiber supplementation nor the IP_6 treatment had any significant adverse effects on the rats' mineral status.

Thanks (but no thanks) to the rather unfair negative publicity IP_6 as phytic acid had received in the decades past. Aside from the above study in my lab, there are many others that have shown beyond reasonable doubt that IP_6 is safe and long-term administration does *not* affect the mineral status of the experimental animals. Without belaboring the issue, I shall refer you to one of the latest studies done in humans: W. Krittaphol and colleagues from the University of Otago in New Zealand reported in the November – December 2006 issue of the *International Journal of Food Sciences* (vol 57, pages 520-527, 2006) on a study performed in school children in Ubon Ratchathani province of Northeast Thailand. Diet composites were analyzed for zinc, iron calcium, IP_5 and IP_6.

"The inositol penta-phosphate (IP5) and hexaphosphate (IP6) levels were so low they were below the detection limit, attributed in part to leaching of water-soluble potassium and magnesium phytate from glutinous rice after soaking overnight before cooking. <u>Clearly, phytate will not compromise mineral absorption from these diets</u> (underline added). Instead, low zinc intakes are probably primarily responsible for the low zinc status of these children. In contrast, altho-

ugh intakes of dietary iron appear low, the pre-valence of biochemical iron deficiency was also low, suggesting that iron absorption may have been higher than previously assumed." – Krittaphol et al. 2006.

To summarize, these studies therefore suggest that a) IP$_6$ is safe and so is diet rich in IP$_6$, and b) epidemiological, laboratory and clinical studies, all support that IP$_6$ not only has beneficial health effects, but that dietary supplementation with IP$_6$ is more effective than gorging enormous amounts of bran for fighting various diseases.

My Introduction to IP$_6$

I was first introduced to the subject matter of IP$_6$ in the summer of 1985 by the article of Drs Graf and Eaton – and I was hooked. I read and reread the article several times. Their reference to IP$_6$ as phytate was puzzling to me. I however saw the relationship between IP$_6$ in our diet and the lower phosphorylated forms of Inositol such as IP$_3$ since at the time scientists were just starting to delve into the secrets of the inositol phosphates. For instance, inositol triphosphate (IP$_3$) had recently been discovered then and was attributed to the vital function in the transfer of chemical information within our cells. I wanted to adhere to the specific syntax that had been created to name the inositol phosphates so that a relationship between IP_6 in our diet (also in the soil) and the inositol phosphates including IP_6 within our cells could be apparent [but, we did not know then that IP_6 was in our cell, it was only my logical assumption]. I therefore proceeded to coin the term IP_6 for inositol hexaphosphate, instead of phytate or worse phytic acid. Thinking of IP_6 as a single compound within a larger family of inositol phosphates set the stage for the formulation of several hypotheses and for a series of lab experiments over the next few years. It also paved the way for numerous discoveries about the health benefits associated with this unique substance – now a product.

IP₆ is found everywhere

Though the discovery of IP_6 dates back to 1855, it is only during the last two decades or so that we have realized its existence in not just plants, but also animals. In virtually all mammalian (and thus also in human) cells, IP_6 regulates vital functions; heart, brain and skeletal muscles contain the highest concentrations.

Inositol molecules can be found within the cell membranes. Cell membranes serve not only to protect our cells, but they also regulate the flow of nutrients and the shuttling of waste products in and out of the cells. Among the membranes' constituents are molecules called phospholipids, which consist of essential fats and the mineral phosphorrus. One of these phospholipids is phosphatidyl-inositol.

When the cell membranes interact with various hormones, neurotransmitters, or with other chemical substances, inositol compounds break off together with a varying number of phosphorus groups. Among the inositol phosphates, we find IP$_6$, IP$_5$, IP$_4$, IP$_3$, IP$_2$ and IP$_1$. More recently, pyrophosphates of Inositol such as IP$_7$ and IP$_8$ have been discovered within our cells and these seem to have functions akin to IP$_6$. IP$_3$ - the most popular amongst cell biologists and inositol phosphate researchers till now, has earned its place owing to its crucial role in regulating various cell functions by influencing cellular calcium metabolism.

IP$_6$ can be involved in two vital chemical processes that continue to intrigue biochemists and cell biologists. I am referring to:

- Phosphorylation, a chemical process whereby phosphate groups are *added* to a molecule;

- Dephosphorylation, a process that *removes* phosphate groups from a molecule.

The molecule of interest here is of course inositol which may be attached to anywhere from one to six (or more as in pyrophosphates) phosphate groups.

In what ways do phosphorylation and dephosphorylation affect cell function? What we know is that those inositol phosphates act as messengers between individual cells. The moment one of these IP molecules comes in contact with a cell structure, a chemical message is transferred. This can occur in one of two ways:

- The inositol phosphates bind to the outside of cell membranes and then impact cell processes through the membrane;

- The inositol phosphates act directly inside the cells themselves.

It is a well-established fact that inositol 1, 4, 5-tri-phosphate (IP$_3$) can activate a host of cell func-tions. (As an aside, the three numbers in IP$_3$'s name correspond to the carbon atoms on the ino-sitol molecule to which phosphate groups are att-ached (the inositol molecule contains six carbon atoms).

What functions are controlled by the higher forms of inositol phosphates? IP$_5$ (inositol 1, 3, 4, 5, 6-pentasphosphate) and IP$_6$ represent the bulk of the inositol phosphates found within mammalians cells. In fact, virtually every mammalian cell con-tains these inositol phosphates; interestingly, they are found in far greater quantity than any of the other inositol phosphates discussed above.

Why should IP$_5$ and IP$_6$ be more abundant in the cell? What is nature's purpose behind this? Recent studies may provide some insight into this ques-tion. For instance, it is known that IP$_5$ is involved in regulating avian hemoglobin's ability to absorb and hold oxygen (avian hemoglobin is a vital red blood cell component found in birds). IP$_5$ and IP$_6$ may also be associated with the stimulation of ner-ve cells, as demonstrated by Dr. Menniti and his colleagues in 1993. Both IP$_5$ and IP$_6$ play a very dynamic role within the cell, and in fact to a far greater extent than previously anticipated (in the past, these compounds were thought to be relatively inactive and were thus termed "metabolically lethargic"). That IP_6 is far from lazy is now being increasingly recognized in the form of its active role in mRNA transport, chromatin remodeling, DNA repair, cell proliferation and differentiation, cell death (apoptosis) etc. A detailed review of these functions can be found in a book-chapter I have composed (Shamsuddin, A. M.: Cell signaling properties of inositol hexaphosphate, In: Rimbach G., Fuchs J., and Packer L., editors. *Nutrigenomics: The Role of Oxidants and Antioxidants in Gene Expression.* CRC Press, Taylor & Francis Group. Boca Raton, Florida, USA. 2005 pp 397-42).

In recent days IP_7 and IP_8 - inositol pyrophosphates have also been detected within our cells. In the 17 December 2004 issue of the journal *Science* (volume 306 #5704, pages 2101-2105) Dr. Saiardi and others at Professor Solomon Snyder's lab at the Johns Hopkins University in Baltimore reported that by using radiolabeled IP_7, they detected phosphorylation of multiple eukaryotic proteins as well as phosphorylation of endogenous proteins by endogenous IP_6 in yeast. It appeared that phosphorylation by IP_7 is non-enzymatic and thus may represent a novel intracellular signaling mechanism, establishing the role of IP_7 as a signal transducer as well. Earlier studies also from Professor Snyder's lab showed that IP_7 may mediate chemotaxis (chemically attracting other cells) in yeasts.

Scientific interest in IP_6 has waxed and waned ever since it was discovered. Initially, IP_6 became a popular research item chiefly because of the discovery that it served as a primary storage form for phosphorus. Phosphorous is a vital nutrient that is required by all cells and by germinating seeds. Phosphorus is a key component of adenosine triphosphate or ATP - perhaps the most important molecule found in cells. ATP is a molecule with the capacity to store energy inside cells. Without ATP, cells would not function and the organism that relies on them would die. This principle holds true for any living organism – be it a plant, an animal, or a human being.

IP_6 supplies the cell with phosphorus, which - as we have seen - is a crucial component of ATP and thus of the cell's energy household. This means IP_6 most likely plays an essential role in maintaining vital cellular energy processes. And how might that be?

Let's look at the energy management of the cell as a rechargeable electrical battery. The chemicals in the battery store the energy which is used (discharged). During the various processes in our cells energy is consumed which is provided by hydrolysis of ATP $\rightarrow$ ADP (adenosine diphosphate); as in the electrical battery, our cellular 'battery' too needs to be recharged; our cells do that by oxidizing glucose during which process ADP is converted back to ATP. It is now known that IP₆ is needed for activation of at least certain ATPase - enzyme that hydrolyzes ATP$\rightarrow$ADP (Hodge *et al* 2011). As in the electrical battery (our cars for example), it is critical that our cellular battery remains constantly charged. I submit that IP₆ by being a storage form of phosphate - a bank, contributes to the health (charged status) of our cellular "battery' by being a constant and reliable source of phosphates.

Phytate - The Bad, IP₆ - The Good!

Over the past 50 years, some researchers, especially in the field of nutrition have been alluding to the fact that the intakes of foods high in IP₆ (phytate) promote mineral deficiencies – phytate the bad! Recently, societies have become more health-conscious and have adopted diets that put more emphasis on plant-based foods (which are high in fiber and in IP_6) – certainly a switch from the more traditional meat and potato diet. Coupled with the availability of IP_6 as a dietary supplement, this has sparked a fresh interest in IP_6's role in mineral balance. Soybeans have been processed into food products that look, smell, and most importantly taste just like meat. A positive side effect of new food products is that they contain substantial amounts of IP_6. I would now like to further elaborate on this topic.

IP_6 has been shown to create chemical complexes – called chelates – with a wide range of minerals that are known to be important for a balanced nutrition. These minerals range from calcium to zinc. The term chelate is derived from the Greek word '*chele*' for claw. The IP_6 molecule - when it chelates minerals - literally creates a claw or basketlike structure that holds the above-mentioned minerals.

In vitro, that is to say in the laboratory, IP_6 (inositol hexaphosphoric *acid*) will form complexes with positively charged mineral atoms known as ions. The following ions are listed in decreasing order of their binding (i.e., chelating) ability: Copper

(Cu), zinc (Zn), cobalt (Co), manganese (Mn), iron (Fe), and calcium (Ca).

Because of its ability to chelate, it has been widely believed that IP_6 would actually *reduce* the bio-availability of these minerals in our diet. Given the belief that chelation prevents these minerals from being used effectively by the body, most of the scientific interest was focused on IP_6's potentially inhibiting impacts on mineral absorption. But can this be substantiated?

When attempting to determine a substance's pro-perties, the standard course of action is to render it in its purest possible form before commencing a study. It is noteworthy that almost all - if not all of the studies that concluded IP_6 had an inhibitory effect (on, say the absorption of iron) were *not* carried out with IP_6 in its purest form. Instead, such studies were typically performed with diets that included foods known to be rich in IP_6. In other words, pure or isolated compounds were absent in these studies. In the meantime, we know that IP_6 has a tendency to bind to food proteins, and that this predisposes it to decomposition by the enzymes in our intestines. This implies that much less IP_6 will be available to fight cancer or other diseases. Furthermore, the binding of proteins may also hamper IP_6's absorption from the stomach.

In contrast, when IP_6 is ingested in a pure form, it binds far less to protein and is therefore more readily available to our cells, and in larger amounts.

Coming back to chelation, yes, inositol hexaphosphoric *acid* can chelate minerals in the test tube in the laboratory setting; but please keep in mind that inositol hexaphosphoric *acid* does not exist in nature and I sincerely hope that no one is marketing it as a dietary supplement, it would be criminal! *No*, the naturally occurring salts of inositol hexaphosphate (sold as the dietary supplements) do not cause the chelation in a normal individual (in conditions of excess iron or copper, the supplement has been found to chelate them to the benefit of the consumer!); they already are attached with the minerals calcium and magnesium! In any event, to reassure you, time and time again, I shall come back to this issue and refer to the results of various studies showing that IP_6 does not cause any adverse reaction insofar as mineral absorption is concerned.

CHAPTER 5

CANCER
PREVENTION BY
IP$_6$ + INOSITOL

Cancer - a Global Problem

Worldwide, some 6.6 million people die of cancer
every year; in the year 2008 there were 12.7 million (12,662,554 to be exact!) new cases of cancer
globally. The number of new victims is estimated

to go up by 69% in 2030; Asia, Latin America and Africa leading the increases by 75%, 86% and 87% respectively. Of the 12.7 million new cases, at 6.09 million Asia had the lion-share, followed by Europe (3.2 million), North America (1.6 million), Latin America and the Caribbean (906,008), and Africa at 681,094 (O'Callaghan 2011). In the United States alone, an estimated 560,000 people succumb to the disease annually; in addition, almost 1.4 million new cases are diagnosed every year. It is therefore no exaggeration to state that cancer is a major public health problem.

The earliest known cases of cancer were described around 2625 B.C.E. by the ancient Egyptian physician Imhotep; the 45th of his teaching cases were about "bulging tumors of the breast" and as to the treatment he offered "none" (Mukherjee 2010, Pederson 2011). In contrast to Imhotep, 4600+ years later, though modern physicians and surgeons are offering some treatment, we are still a long way from curing the disease. Some 40 years ago, in December 1971, US President Richard M. Nixon declared "war on cancer" and since that time, an enormous amount of money (approximately US$90 billion) has been spent by the US government, let alone the private sector in an endeavor to learn about the biology, treatment and prevention of this disease (Marshall E *Science* 331: 1540, 2011)[1]. From time to time, the 'generals' leading the war – those bosses engaged in the field of cancer research – report exciting new gains they achieved in the battlefield. But overall, despite continued efforts and a great deal of optimism, we are simply not yet in a position to declare victory; we have not won the war against this disease, unfortunately not yet!

Research organizations, such as the *National Cancer Institute* and the *American Cancer Society* – just to name two - often make decision as to the next moves in the ongoing battle against cancer. It is at such organizations that decision-makers set the new targets and provide support for the scientific community - all in an effort to develop "silver bullets" that might serve to attack cancer cells. The scientists working in the field generally approve of this approach given that it funds their research and follow the leaders not unlike the foot-soldiers in the battlefield following their commanders.

Among the newest developments in the fight against cancer are therapies that use monoclonal anti-

---

[1] Apparently, the phrase "war on cancer" has been the product of news reports, there was never an official declaration (Marshall E *Science* 331: 1540, 2011)

bodies to target cancer cells. Another example is the use of interleukins and interferon; these give a boost to the immune system and help it control the spread of cancer. And then there is gene therapy. Although we have not been able to vanquish the menace of cancer, such therapies (and the scientists responsible for their development) often receive much recognition and acclaim in the popular media.

In stark contrast, those research efforts that are also innovative, yet do not follow in the footsteps of conventional, mainstream approaches (i.e., that don't necessarily focus on new cancer drugs or radiation therapies) appear to be far less appreciated and typically remain underfunded. While not following the *status quo*, such research – which is typically carried out by independent scientists – should not be dismissed. It too advances the cause, results in new therapies, and brings new hope. I include my own research in this category.

The eminent molecular biologist Dr. Arthur Kornberg stated in the journal *Science* (1997):

"A common __illusion__ is that strategic objectives are necessary to discover the cure for cancer and AIDS and that groups of sufficient size needs to

be mobilized for wars and crusades against these enemies. <u>Nothing could be more misguided</u> [underlines mine]. In the history of triumphs in medical research such wars and crusades have invariably failed because they lacked the necessary weapons – the essential knowledge of basic life processes. Instead, some of the major advances – X-rays, penicillin, polio vaccine, and genetic engineering – have come from the efforts of individual scientists to understand Nature..."

Based on my personal research, what have I learned about IP₆, inositol and cancer?

Before I discuss details of my own research - which was carried out both on animals and directly on human cancer cells – let me share my excitement about the great benefits and safety I see in using inositol to treat humans. In fact, I see the combination of IP₆+inositol as the silver bullet that gives cancer a one two punch! As a wise man once said, "What you find on the road you travel to reach your goal is often just as important as the goal itself". With that in mind, let us now travel down that road and look at specific research results.

My Initial Approach

I asked the question what role IP_6 and inositol play in the prevention of cancer. To address the topic, I had to formulate experiments that would yield useful answers.

Typically, experiments devised to study the effects of nutrition on cancer involve the addition of a specific nutrient – IP_6 in this particular instance – to food. My own experience in the field of pharmacology persuaded me that it would be far more appropriate to add IP_6 to the drinking water instead. In this way, the experimental animals could absorb the IP_6 more readily. The rats involved in lab experiments cannot be given pure supplements; they cannot be fed with IP_6 in tablet or capsule form. Furthermore, as stated, I did not want to add IP_6 to their food because I believed this would interfere with the rate at which IP_6 would be absorbed. In order to overcome this dilemma, I decided to add IP_6 to the rats' drinking water - an approach roughly akin to persuading humans to take oral supplements with their water (in between meals). My initial thought was that I should try this method myself before feeding an IP_6 solution to the rats. Given that inositol is chemically a sugar, this was no problem; it tasted just fine. I therefore surmised that the rats would like it, too.

My first challenge was to formulate a solution the rats would actually drink. I discovered that they would only consume the liquid at concentrations no greater than 5%. After some tinkering I had determined that the best dose was 2% IP_6 or less. This concentration enabled the rats to consume their normal daily quantity of water. If we compare this amount to a human weighing 70 kg, the IP_6 solution given to the rats would correspond roughly to one to two grams (i.e., 1000 to 2000 mg) of IP_6 taken orally.

In our experiments, I wanted to establish how effective IP_6 is in fighting different tumors in various animal species and to keep matters simple, I decided to first test IP_6 alone and then IP_6+ inositol. For this purpose, we tested two carcinogens known to cause colon cancer: Azoxymethane and 1, 2-dimethylhydrazine. These carcinogens were used on the rats and on the mice respectively.

Two weeks prior to the administration of the carcinogens, the rats began receiving the IP_6 solution. This phase of the experiment is called the preinitiation phase; it is designed to test if IP_6 can *prevent* the earliest process of cancer formation; in other words, whether a treatment with IP₆ would cancel out the effects of the carcinogens. Furthermore, since I could not predict the outcome with certainty, I wanted to give the treatment a certain amount of time to start working.

Six months into the experiment, we found that the average number of tumors developed by the control rats (who were not given any IP₆) was 4.6 per animal. In contrast, the rats treated with IP₆ showed an average of 3 tumors per animal. Furthermore, the tumors produced by those rats that had received IP₆ were approximately two thirds smaller. And the differences were statistically significant.

Early on in the experiments, I witnessed a further effect of IP₆. It concerned the rats that had been treated with IP₆ yet had still developed some tumors. In these animals, we measured the rate of cell division of colon cells that had remained without tumors (i.e., that were non-tumorous). It was discovered that the rate of cell division in these colon cells was very similar to the rate of cell division found in the healthy control animals! What this means is that IP₆ was found to have a regulatory function that serves to normalize (i.e., mitigate) the abnormal increase in cell division (as induced by the carcinogens). We also discovered that animals that had received IP_6 but not the carcinogens showed normal rates of cell division. This finding strongly indicate that IP_6 can actually normalize (i.e., bring down to normal levels) the rate of cell division in cells that already show abnormally increased cell growth rate (which is a characteristic stage during the formation of cancer). It also demonstrated that IP_6 however does not impact the normal rate of cell division found in healthy animals. Subsequent studies proved this in human cell lines as well. Most noteworthy, the results were statistically significant; in other words, this was the kind of result that is scientifically valid.

If you are interested in further details regarding these experiments, please consult my research publications for the years 1988, 1989, and 1990 (refer to the Bibliography).

But why were the tumors in the animals treated with IP_6 smaller? Does this mean that IP_6 might be effective even in situations where a cancer is already established (during the so-called post-initiation phase)? To follow up on this finding, we gave IP_6 as early as two weeks after, and as late as five months *after* the administration of the carcinogens.

Even in those animals subjected to a carcinogen treatment two weeks, or five months *prior* to a treatment with IP_6, my coworkers Ashish Chakaravarthy, Asad Ullah, AlaaEldeen Elsayed and I still found that the IP_6 had inhibited the development of cancer. In this context, please note that because we started IP_6 treatment at a later point (5 months later, as compared to the first experiments done after 2 weeks), I decided to give the rats a higher dose of 2% rather than the 1% in the previous experiment, done so that the cancer does not enjoy an unfair advantage.

Following are some results we found 8 months into the experiment, based on four applications of the carcinogen azoxymethane:

- Only 10% of the animals that had received IP_6 were found to have colon cancer;

- In contrast, 43% of those not receiving IP_6 had developed the cancer.

In our experiments, the animals that had received IP_6 as long as 5 months after the initiation of cancer (i.e., at a point where we anticipated most of the rats would now have the disease) were found to have developed significantly fewer tumors.

Even more importantly, their tumors were smaller compared to the tumors developed by the animals that had not been given IP_6. We conclude that IP_6 has possible therapeutic applications - even for existing cancers.

Table 5-1: Experimental inhibition of colon cancer after five months

Treatment	Tumors / Rat	Mitotic Rate % in non-tumorous area
Carcinogen only. Azoxymethane (AOM)	7.1	2.3
AOM + IP_6	5.2	1.0

Table 5-1 shows some of the data we gathered from our experiments. Specifically, it reports to what extent colon cancer was inhibited by the use of IP_6, as reflected in the decreased number of tumors per animal (i.e., the tumor frequency), and the lower rate of cell division (i.e., the mitotic rate).

Was there a dose-dependent relationship between the amount of IP_6 and the incidence of large intestinal cancer? Put differently, could this cancer be further reduced if more IP_6 was given? In an effort to answer this question, in 1990 Asad Ullah and I proceeded to test the doses of IP_6 ranging from as low as 0.1% to as high as 1%. (For comparative purposes, in a 70-kg human, the equivalent oral doses would range between 100 mg and 1000 mg/day).

We found a reduced prevalence of tumors as the dosage of IP_6 was stepped up. Using a dose of 1% IP_6, at the end of the 44-week experiment, results also showed a dose-related reduction in the prevalence of tumors by 52.2%.

I had developed a hypothesis about IP_6's positive action against cancer. As discussed in the previous chapter, IP_6 is subject to dephosphorylation, a process whereby it can be converted into IP_{1-5}. I had postulated that IP_6 could enter into the inositol phosphate pool found inside cells. Once inside a cell, it might then be converted into IP_3 and serve to suppress tumors by virtue of the action of the lower-numbered inositol phosphates. Already in 1988, I had hypothesized that the addition of inositol to IP_6 could enhance IP_6's cancer fighting powers. (Inositol has been known to be a safe, natural carbohydrate from which IP_6 is formed). We knew that there are enzymes in the body that can remove the phosphates from IP_6 – dephosphorylation (caused by phosphatases specifically phytase), and enzymes who can add phosphates to inositol resulting in formation of IP_{1-6} (now IP_{7-8} as well) called kinases. So why shouldn't we get more of IP_3 in our body as per the following hypothetical reaction if we took IP_6+inositol together?

$$IP_6 + inositol = 2\ IP_3$$

Recall that IP_3 is the molecule that is crucial for a large variety of cellular function in almost all, if not all mammalian cells. Thus, the anticancer capabilities of the inositol phosphates should be observable in various different cells and organs.

My working hypotheses were:

1. IP_6 works through the lower inositol phosphates (IP_{1-5} but most likely IP_3) in the intracellular inositol phosphate pool

2. Addition of inositol may enhance the anti-cancer action of IP_6

3. Since the inositol phosphates are in all mammalian cells and the cells all

share a common pathway of cell division as well as cell signaling, the anti-cancer action of IP_6 ± inositol should be visible in different cancers and in different species

By the end of 1987, I had succeeded in proving the following:

- IP_6 was shown to have prevented colon cancer in rats and in mice (part of Hypothesis III);

- Inositol also has cancer-inhibiting effects; however, by itself it is not as effective as IP_6;

- IP_6 and inositol work in a synergistic union – in other words, they enhance each other when present together (Hypothesis II); additionally

- Both IP_6 and inositol stimulated immune cells, the combination of IP_6+inositol was by far much better in boosting the immune system. The underlying mechanism is the stimulation of NK cells (<u>n</u>atural <u>k</u>iller cells, specialized immune system cells with the

capacity to fight cancer); bonus point on
Hypothesis II!

Having proven the second and the third (in part)
hypotheses, my co-workers and I set out to test the
first and the remainder of the third: does IP_6 work
through the lower inositol phosphates and would
IP_6+Inositol be a broad spectrum anti-cancer agent
– effective against a variety of cancers, and not just
in rats and mice but also in humans?

For that we treated K-562 *human* erythroleukemia cells with IP_6. These are human blood cancer
cells that lose the ability to produce hemoglobin.
Our reasoning for selecting these human leukemia cells was that *if* IP_6 could indeed "normalize"
these (aberrant) cells, they would then be able to
manufacture hemoglobin (which is a typical function of red blood cells) an effect we could easily
measure – quantitation is an objective evaluation.
We found that those cells that had been treated
with IP_6 showed higher levels of hemoglobin; on
the other hand, this was not the case for the untreated K–562 cells. The findings implied that the
treated cells had reverted back to a more normal
(or mature) state and behaving normally, a process
called "differentiation". Concomitant to this increased differentiation was reduction in the rate of

increased cell growth as we have observed in the rats and mice.

But, more to the point was that not only did we demonstrate that IP_6 enters inside the K–562 cells, but we were also able to measure a significant incr- ease (of 41%) in the concentration of IP_3 inside the cells. We also showed that IP_6 is converted to lower forms of inositol once inside cells. Our exp- eriments, as well as those of others, now indicate that IP_6 is rapidly converted to inositol as well as to IP_{1-5}. Thus, supplying an organism with IP_6 will change the quantities of the various inositol phos- phates within its cells. Furthermore, we also estab- lished that there is a correlation between such changes inside the cell and an ensuing reduction in cell division. The growth rate of a cell is influen- ced by its intracellular level of calcium. IP_6 may bring *abnormal* cell division to a standstill by trig- gering an increase in the amount of calcium found inside a cell.

Numerous studies have indicated that an increase in calcium concentration can result in cell division; however, our data showed just the opposite: A reduction in cell division! How can we explain this apparent contradiction? Typically, IP_3 promotes cell division. But why addition of inositol and IP_6

with resultant increased intracellular IP$_3$ would lower the rate of cell division and by extension the risk of developing cancer? Is it some sort of negative feedback control observed commonly in biological systems? At this point the answer is a simple "I don't know!"

"The only knowledge I have is that I have no knowledge" ...Socrates

To add to the conundrum, in 1997, two of my associates – Dr. Katherine E. Cole and Mary Smith – demonstrated that an addition of IP$_6$ to human colon tumor cells prompted a three- to fourfold rise in calcium within those cells - all in the time span of 10 seconds! Such a rapid, dramatic increase in the calcium concentration would seem to indicate that IP$_6$ exerts some kind of action on the cells' receptors. But the increased intracellular calcium now reconfirmed in yet another human cell type (previous study on K-562 erythroleukemia cells) with *reduced* cell division goes contrary to the generally accepted principle that increased intracellular calcium triggers cell division! Be that as it may, in this particular instance, evidence suggests that IP$_6$ may block certain growth receptors without which cancer cells fail to grow and multiply.

At a later time, we found that this conjecture proved to be correct! Inositol does indeed boost IP_6's ability to restrain cell division, as well as its anti-tumor effect *in vivo* (i.e. in the living body). When we added inositol to the IP_6, we found a statistically significant enhancement in the suppression of cell proliferation, and of colorectal cancer.

These studies were expanded to experimental models of mammary cancer and metastatic tumors by my colleague Dr. Ivana Vucenik. Motivated by the compelling therapeutic possibilities these experiments had brought to light, Dr. Kosaku Sakamoto, a surgeon from Gunma University in Japan who left his lucrative practice of surgery and applied himself tirelessly in my laboratory for two years, without financial compensation!

In pioneering works such as this, soon we needed confirmation by others to assure us that we are in the right track...these all seem *"too good to be true!"* What about other researchers? Has their work with IP_6 yielded similar results? Though for a while I was the only one travelling this path [many, many thanks to the dedication and loyalty of my associates who believed in my outlandish ideas], I was so pleased to read Dr. Theresa Pretlow's paper from Case Western Reserve University in

Cleveland, Ohio. Five [long] years since our report in 1987 (Elsayed *et al*) she wrote:

"The incidence of tumors in F344 rats treated with AOM without phytate was 83% (10/12) compared to 25% (3/12) in rats treated with AOM plus phytate [IP6]…" -T. P. Pretlow et al. (1992).

In October 1992, Dr. Pretlow's research group reported their results at the *Third Annual Conference on Nutrition and Cancer* held by the *American Institute for Cancer Research* in McLean, Virginia. Not only was IP₆ effective in inhibiting colon cancer, it was also shown to do so, far better than other chemopreventive agents (such as selenium, for example). An article that dealt with this research topic was published in 1994 in *Advances of Experimental Medicine and Biology* entitled: "Colon Carcinogenesis is inhibited *more effectively by phytate* [italics mine] than by Selenium in F344 rats given 30 mg per kilogram azoxymethane."[2]

---

[2] Dr. Pretlow's lab initially failed to confirm our findings as they had added IP₆ to the feed (as opposed to drinking water); following our discussion in a scientific meeting the study was reproduced obtaining results similar to ours.

Equally compelling is that IP$_6$'s anti-tumor (anti-neoplastic) action is probably not restricted to the colon. We and others have demonstrated this. One thing that must however be taken into consideration when reviewing these data is that the method of supplying the IP$_6$ varied among some of the experiments. For instance, when IP$_6$ was given as bran (i.e., as phytate), one could reasonably expect that it would be biologically less active than if it had been supplied in its pure form (as IP$_6$ or as IP$_6$+inositol). As shown earlier, the addition of IP$_6$ to food tends to reduce its efficacy due to IP$_6$'s tendency to form complexes with food proteins. This may explain the slightly differing results reported by the various investigators at least in the early papers.

IP₆ at Work Inside Our Cells

Unfortunately, we did not then know the precise pathways by means of which IP$_6$ achieves its demonstrated anti-cancer action. One aspect to consider is that nutritionists and agronomists never really looked very closely at IP$_6$ – at least not for its health benefits. Instead, they were first and foremost preoccupied [perhaps somewhat obsessed may be] with the unfounded fear of IP$_6$'s possible "toxic" effects – and much of that research was based on outdated and otherwise inadequate data dealing with 'phytate's mineral chelating' capacity [I had encountered aggressive not just verbal comments, but also physical gestures from otherwise gentle and polite octogenarian opponents in scientific meetings!].

It is my humble opinion that the lack of studies on IP₆'s health benefits stemmed from not having co-operative research efforts between nutritionists, cell biologists, and biochemists. It seems no one wanted to see the big picture! Some scientists ignored IP₆ altogether, a topic addressed by F. S. Menniti and colleagues in 1993. For some time, researchers even believed that organisms could not absorb IP₆; others thought it simply did not have any beneficial functions to fulfill within the cell. Despite preliminary studies carried out by Drs. Nahapetian and Young from Shiraz University in Iran and Massachusetts Institute of Technology (MIT) in Cambridge, USA, back in 1980; some scientists even ignored the evidence that IP₆ is actually absorbed [even their MIT affiliation did not sway them!]. Equally brushed aside was early research that indicated IP₆ was present in cells and that various mechanisms exist to shuttle IP₆ molecules across cell membranes!

Today, with cancer recognized as a major public health issue, we should strive to further our understanding of the mechanisms that underpin IP_6's dramatic anticancer effects. My laboratory experiments have clearly demonstrated that IP_6 is readily absorbed from the stomach and from the upper small intestine of rats, and furthermore, that it is subsequently distributed to various organs – as quickly as one hour after being administered (Sakamoto *et al* 1993). Using radioactive tracers, we were able to show that inositols, as well as combinations of inositol + phosphate (IP_{1-6}) – were present in the lining of the stomach. Inositol and IP_1 were found in the urine and blood plasma. The discovery of this molecule with fewer phosphate groups in such areas of the body indicates that these compounds are rapidly metabolized. The fact that we found IP_6 in the stomach lining is an indication that it must have been transported into the cells' interior and undergone rapid dephosphorylation.

We have demonstrated that not only exogenously given IP_6 is quickly absorbed from the gastrointestinal tract, but it also is rapidly taken up by malignant cells; orally administered IP_6 can reach target tumor tissue distant from the gastrointestinal tract.

By analyzing the absorption, intracellular distribution and metabolism of IP_6 in HT-29 human colon cancer cell line and cells of hematopoietic lineage (K-562 human erythroleukemia and YAC-1 mouse lymphoma cells), we have found that exogenous IP_6 is rapidly taken up by these cells, transported intracellularly by the mechanisms involving pinocytosis and/or receptor-mediated endocytosis and dephosphorylated into inositol phosphates with fewer phosphate groups. Likewise, when MCF-7 human breast cancer cells were incubated with radiolabeled IP_6 as early as 1 min after incubation 3.1% of IP_6-associated radioactivity was taken up by MCF-7 cells and 9.5% after 1 h. Chromatographic analysis showed that 58% of the absorbed radioactivity was in IP_6. However, IP_4 seemed to be a predominant metabolite of IP_6, which possibly might have important role in its anticancer activity in these cells. To summarize, these data indicate that the intact IP_6 molecule was transported inside the gastric epithelial cells, wherein it was rapidly dephosphorylated, and that the metabolism of IP_6 was very rapid. When radiolabeled IP_6 was given *via* oral gavage to rats bearing mammary tumors, a substantial amount of radioactivity (19.7% of all radioactivity recovered in collected tissues) was found in tumor tissue as early as 1 h after administration. This suggests that

IP_6 goes directly and accumulates preferentially in tumor sites distant from the gastrointestinal tract.

As you can imagine, this too was an "outrageous" finding. That is because it has been [and continues to be the belief amongst a few diehards] that IP_6, a highly charged and highly hydrophilic molecule, cannot pass the plasma membrane passively and enter the cells. Fortunately, in a subsequent public-cation in the December 2002 issue of the journal *Carcinogenesis* (volume 23: pages 2031-2041, 2002), Dr. Sandra Ferry then working at Professor Hirata's laboratory in Kyushu University, Japan provided confirmation to our data and our original hypothesis that the externally applied IP_6 enters the cell followed by dephosphorylation.

"These results revealed that extracellularly app-lied InsP6 directly activates the apoptotic machi-nery as well as inhibits the cell survival signaling, probably by the intracellular delivery followed by a de-phosphorylation."

They also demonstrated that IP_6 is internalized into the cells by the process of pinocytosis. Using new-er technologies, such as inductively coupled plas-ma atomic emission spectrometry (ICP-AES), Professor Grases and his coworkers (2001) in Spain were able to identify IP_6 in human urine and plasma and detect IP_5 and its less-phosphorylated forms (IP_{3-5}) in mammalian cells and in body fluids, as they occur naturally; the peak plasma value of IP_6 is reached at 4 hours after an oral dose.

Pharmacokinetics in a mouse model carrying xeno-transplanted human breast cancer shows that the plasma concentration of IP_6 peaked at 5 minutes after intravenous injection and remained detectable for 45 minutes. Liver IP_6 concentration was 10-fold higher than that in the plasma, whereas the levels in other tissues were same as the plasma. Interestingly, only inositol was detected in the tumor xenografts. In contrast to intravenous administration, IP_6 was detected only in the liver following oral intake, all other organs showed the presence of inositol. Since the ability to dephosphorylate IP_6 varies widely between different species (rat small intestine has a 30-fold higher phytase level than human, Iqbal *et al 1994*), pharmacokinetics data from *oral* administration of IP_6 in rodents may not apply to the human.

IP_6 may form complexes with a variety of proteins and other molecules. When this occurs, we see a slowing of its absorption and metabolic activation. This is particularly the case when IP_6 is ingested solely as part of a diet (i.e., eaten together with other food components). On the other hand, an oral administration of IP_6 in its pure form is expected to be more effective. A comparison of various studies on the topic underscore this notion. For example, when comparatively smaller amounts of IP_6 were administered every second day (Vucenik *et al.*, 1992), similar success rates in terms of tumor inhibition were noted as compared to other studies, where greater amounts of IP_6 were mixed in with the diet (Jariwalla et al., 1988). In 1991, Hirose and colleagues came to similar conclusions: In their work, they did not see a statistically significant inhibition of colon tumors from dietary IP_6; however, they did report a modest inhibition of the development of liver and pancreatic tumors.

By this time you must be tempted to ask the question: So if IP_6 is that great why is the US National Cancer Institute (NCI) not paying any attention? It seems that they did, and did not. Supported by several National Cancer Institute contracts, in the February 1, 1995 *Cancer Research* (volume 55: pages 537-543) paper, Dr. Julia Arnold from *ManTech Environmental Technology*, Research Triangle Park, North Carolina and her colleague Dr. Vernon Steele from the Chemoprevention Branch of the Division of Cancer Prevention and Control of NCI, Bethesda, Maryland reported on the finding of their evaluation of 99 different chemopreventive agents of interest in a Rat Tracheal Epithelial Transformation assay. IP_6 (IHP in their abbreviation) showed a 78% inhibition (Table 2 in page 541). Why that was not pursued, is a question you will have to ask the scientists. I had personally approached NCI both directly and indirectly through a US Congressman and a Senator in vain. A description of that ordeal can be found in the book by Drs. Kim Vanderlinden and Ivana Vucenik http://ip-6.net/files/77513690.pdf

CHAPTER 6

CANCER TREATMENT BY IP$_6$+INOSITOL

Experimental Therapy in the Laboratory

One of our lab experiments had clearly demonstrated that an IP$_6$ treatment begun as late as 5 months after cancer initiation was still effective in containing colorectal cancer. This very exciting result led us to the logical question: Could IP$_6$ also be used to treat already existing cancers? In other words, we thought that the application of IP_6 was perhaps not limited solely to preventing the development of cancers. We already knew from previous experiments that IP_6 normalizes the rate of cell division. But, could it really shrink a pre-existing tumor?!

Experimental Model of Metastatic Cancer

Both early-stage and well-established cancers are characterized by an increase in the number of cells. Based on this knowledge, we planned new laboratory studies where we would test the therapeutic properties of IP_6; this was done on mice that already had tumors. Tumors were developed in the animals by injecting them with cancerous mouse fibrosarcoma (FSA–1) cells under the skin. A fibrosarcoma is a cancerous tumor that consists of fibrous connective tissue. One of the reasons to choose these particular cancer cells was to further validate my Hypothesis III that IP_6+Inositol is a broad-spectrum anticancer agent effective against different types of cancers. As opposed to the common cancers of lung, colon, breast, stomach, ovary etc., that are of epithelial origin, fibrosarcomas albeit less common, are of *non*-epithelial origin from mesenchymal tissues. Another reason to decide on this model is to take the studies to the next step: with time cancer cells spread to distant organs, a process called metastasis that often results in the patients' demise. Thus, FSA-1 model being a metastatic one served our purpose to both further validate my Hypothesis III and expand the scope of our investigation towards eventual human use.

In our experiment, when we injected the FSA–1 cells intravenously, we found that the tumors later had spread to the mice's lungs. Having injected the mice with IP_6 every second day, we found a statistically significant inhibition of tumor sizes, as well as an improvement of the animals' survival time (in comparison to those animals that had not received any IP_6). And the combination of IP_6 + inositol yielded the best results. The dose of IP_6 the mice had been injected with was 0.25% - for a 70-kg human, an equivalent dose would be roughly 125 to 250 mg of IP_6. But please, don't rush to inject IP_6 as human trials of injection are yet to be performed.

In 1992, we reported in the journal *Cancer Letters* (Vucenik *et al.*, 1992) that the mice treated with IP_6 showed a significant reduction in the number of tumors that had spread to their lungs (i.e., fewer metastatic lung colonies).

A general summary of the findings from this experiment is that IP_6 not only serves to prevent cancer, it also shows a pronounced anticancer effect even when the disease is already established. Furthermore, this inhibiting effect was seen even when a cancer had already spread to other areas of the body. The experiments further illustrate that an ***uninterrupted treatment with IP₆ is imperative*** in view of achieving the highest possible anticancer effect. In an endeavor to pave the way for future clinical trials in humans, we also studied how safe an administration of IP_6 would be. We found IP_6 to be totally nontoxic - even over the lifetime of the animals. I have been religiously taking it since my patented formulation (IP_6+inositol) has been available in 1998; I am happy to report that I have not had flu or even an attack of common cold since then!

In 1988, Dr. Jariwalla and his colleagues then at the Linus Pauling Institute in California carried out an experiment comparable to the one we performed and which was discussed before, except that rats were used instead of mice. What differentiates their experiment however is that they used a much higher dose of IP$_6$ and IP$_6$ was not given in a pure form in water as we did, but added to the animals' diets. I have already discussed that IP$_6$ may bind with dietary proteins and thereby reduce its bio-availability. On the other hand, supplying IP$_6$ in a pure form ensures that it will be absorbed to a much greater extent, resulting in more pronounced health effects. Just as we had discovered in our experiments, Dr. Jariwalla's studies also produced no adverse health effects (i.e., they found no evidence of toxicity) from the use of IP$_6$. Furthermore, study results pointed to the possibility that IP$_6$ may contribute beneficially toward lower cholesterol levels and a reduced buildup of triglycerides

Cancer Cell Lines

Cancer cell lines consist of populations of cancer cells that are removed from actual tumors and then cultured (i.e., maintained) in a lab setting. In my lab, *in vitro* studies have been carried out on such cancer cell lines – originating both from humans and from rodents. Experimental results indicate that IP$_6$ lowers the cell propagation rate of all the cell lines tested. This means that IP$_6$ prevents such cells from multiplying at an aberrant rate. An interesting side note is that when the cells were given an excessive IP_6, they did not exhibit signs of cytotoxicity (i.e., they did not die off due to an overload of IP_6). This finding is in sharp contrast to research with most other anticancer agents, where adverse effects occur on the cells under such circumstances. Rather than showing signs of cytotoxicity in the presence of IP_6, we found that the growth of the malignant (i.e., cancerous) cells was curtailed – the cells matured and then died off.

You probably can't wait to ask the question: was the combination of IP_6+inositol tested and if not why not? You may recall from the previous chapters that inositol is a B-vitamin and is essential for the growth of cells in artificial media and therefore it is not expected to yield a synergistic reaction *in vitro* as seen *in vivo*. However, Schröterová *et al* (2010) at Charles University in Prague, Czech Republic tested three different cell lines derived from human colon cancers of different stages of malignancy with IP_6 with or without Inositol *in vitro* for inhibition of cell growth and induction of apoptosis. Their data show "a clear indication of Ins enhancing the proapoptotic effect of IP6 in all the cells lines studied."

At this point, it would be helpful to further your understanding of cancer cells. Specifically, why it

Growth Inhibition of HT-29 Human Colon Cancer Cells by InsP6

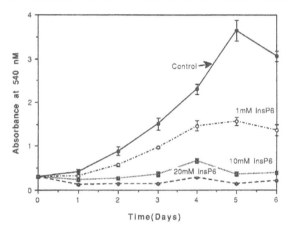

Figure 6-1: Dose-response inhibition of HT-29 Human colon cancer cells by IP₆. Note that at 10mM and 20mM concentrations the cancer cells virtually stopped growing.

is imperative that cancer cells be able to mature? In many cases, cancer cells resemble the types of cells we see in the fetus – in other words, they resemble immature cells that have not specialized such as the cells which we find in the skin or in the heart, for example. Because cancerous cells are immature, they still possess the latent capacity to morph into any number of different cell types.

Another feature of immature cancer cells is that they are far more aggressive, dividing and multiplying more rapidly than ordinary cells. In general, the more immature (de-differentiated to undifferentiated) the cells are, the more aggressive their behavior is. When cancer cells mature, they start to look similar to the differentiated or specialized cells, such as the cells of the liver, the lung, or of the skin - just to name a few. This cell maturing process is typically accompanied by the cells becoming more passive and less aggressive. Cells with a normal phenotype (i.e., appearance) tend to resemble what they were intended to be – skin cells, kidney cells, other specific cell types.

Different cancer cell lines may display characteristic features, such as reduced cell growth and enhanced differentiation – this can occur to such an extent that the cells actually revert back to their normal phenotypes. The neuroblastoma, a highly malignant cancer of nerve cell origin in infants and children may look nothing like nerve cells; but some of them can show areas of differentiation towards looking like nerve and ganglion cells, with accompanying more docile behavior at which point they are called ganglioneuroma. The corollary in the lab is the following: In comparison to their healthy counterpart red blood cells (also

known as erythrocytes), K–562 human erythroleukemia cells tend to be smaller and show a lack of
hemoglobin (the oxygen-transporting molecules
found inside red blood cells). Treatment of K562
cells with IP_6 resulted in a remarkable inhibition of
the growth of these erythroleukemia cells. Only a
few of the cells remained alive 48 hours after initiation of IP_6 treatment. IP_6 treatment reduced the
number of erythroleukemia cells and allowed them
to accumulate hemoglobin; in other words, the
cells became more like mature cells - in this case
the red blood cells (Shamsuddin *et al*, 1992).

What came out of these experiments was the fact
that IP_6 by itself or in combination with inositol is
somehow capable of stimulating or triggering a
process whereby cancerous cells start to adopt normal cell behavior. Let me interpret these findings
by using an analogy of a social situation:

Taming the Cancer Cells

For the sake of argument, let's assume that the cancerous cells are angry youths who subsequently
start a gang (by analogy - the cancer), which then
begins to exhibit destructive behavior, virtually
"eating up" society. Some members of society may

wish to retaliate against this unacceptable behavior by handing out death sentence, trying to eradicate the cancerous cells that are laying waste to the body. However, this extermination attempt may not eradicate the cancerous cells completely. Or, the person attempting the treatment may suffer severe toxic side effects as a result. Then again, society may wish to contemplate less draconian measures, perhaps opting to educate and rehabilitate the misfits instead - in an effort to bring them back into the fold of civilization and return them into productive members of society again.

Enough of the analogies - let's get back to IP₆. It does exactly what was discussed above: Triggering cancer cells to mature and making them behave like normal cells again. This poses an interesting challenge. In the research lab, we can look at tumor cells under a microscope and establish whether they have been vanquished; however, how shall we determine whether or not a treatment with IP₆ has worked and reverted the cancer cells back to normal?

Can it be done in a human? Yes, and this is how: The presence of many cancer cells is associated with a distinct marker otherwise not expressed by healthy cells, or not typically found in normal (healthy) people. This principle applies to many types of cancer, including cancer of the colon, breast, prostate, lungs, pancreas, and others as described in Chapter 1. The marker is Galactose ß-D-Galactose-[1→3]-N-acetyl-galactosamine   or Gal-GalNAc for short.

As described in Chapter 1, healthy cells in normal people do not express the marker Gal-GalNAc. On the other hand, if we were to take a mucus sample from the colon or bronchus of a person afflicted with cancer, the marker would be expressed (I discussed this topic extensively in my 1996 article in *Anticancer Research*). As reviewed in Chapter 1, I had developed a very simple test that can be used to detect Gal-GalNAc, and - by extension - the presence of cancers of the colon, lung, breast etc. Assume that sometime in the past, a rectal mucus sample was taken from a patient with colon cancer (or coughed-up sputum sample or nipple aspirate for lung or breast cancer respectively), and that this sample tested positive for Gal-GalNAc – i.e., the cancer was discovered. Assume the cancer was then surgically removed. It is a well-known fact that patients who have undergone such an operation are now at much higher risk of developing a second cancer - in the same region - at a later point in time. What screening tests are available to monitor the potential reoccurrence (relapse) of the cancer? An unpleasant surprise could be avoided by periodically (re)testing for the marker Gal-GalNAc. For a person who showed a prior positive result for Gal-GalNAc, a negative result at a later time would be a good indication that he/she was currently free of the cancer. If a treatment with IP_6+Inositol is indeed able to reduce the risk of cancer and to prevent its formation (or recurrence), would it not be advantageous if IP_6 could at the same time suppress the expression of Gal-Gal-NAc? If it did, we could then possibly monitor the effect.

Auspiciously, that is not just wishful thinking! With the intent of testing that assumption, we carried out an experiment using an HT–29 human colon cancer cell line. A highly-motivated summer student who came to my lab in 1992 Giridhar Ventkatraman told me that he would like to work simultaneously on two projects, both IP_6 and Gal-GalNAc. This got me thinking: What would happen if IP_6 could indeed suppress Gal-GalNAc in this cell line? Gal-GalNAc is expressed by HT–29, and the marker is located within the mucus of these cells. Supervising him in my lab at the time was Dr. Kosaku Sakamoto – the surgeon from Gunma University in Japan who had left his own, very successful practice of Surgery to apply himself in my lab for two years, all without drawing a salary!

Based on the experiments we carried out together in the summer of that year, we were able to establish that IP_6 suppresses proliferation of HT-29 colon cancer cell line; furthermore, IP_6 also inhibited the expression of the tumor marker Gal-GalNAc to a substantial extent. Even though the cells still continued to produce mucus (which is an indication of their maturity), the majority showed no expression of the tumor marker at all (Sakamoto *et al*, 1993). This implies that while IP_6 impedes the activity of the cancerous cell, it still allows the cells to function normally (and in this case - to produce mucus). In other words, IP_6 permits the human colon cancer cells to mature so that they again resemble normal cells - both in structural and in behavioral (functional) terms. We can also monitor the efficacy of therapy and along with the proper marker follow-up the patient more effectively as has been done in the Croatian study (Vucenik *et al* 2001) cited in Chapter 1.

At a later point, I was also fortunate to have been joined by Dr. Guang-Yu Yang from China Medical University in Shenyang (now a Professor of Pathology at the Northwestern University in Chicago, Illinois in USA), who also contributed to this research. He too was able to independently corroborate our findings that IP$_6$ causes cancerous cells to be normalized and thus fail to express the tumor markers (Yang & Shamsuddin, 1995).

In summary, testing for the marker Gal-GalNAc could be used to establish how well IP$_6$ fights cancer. The test may also serve to determine how effective other anticancer agents are in prompting cells to mature and to differentiate.

Which Types of Cancers can be treated with IP$_6$?

A frequently-used gauge that gives an indication about a drug's or other substance's effectiveness is the so-called inhibitory concentration (IC). When we see a 50% inhibition of cell numbers, we call this the IC$_{50}$ level. As you can well imagine, the dose or concentration that is needed in order to induce the IC$_{50}$ level will vary greatly for different types of cells or cell lines and for different agents. For instance, we know that:

- The cells of a blood-cell forming (i.e., hematopoietic) line show a great sensitivity to

IP$_6$. Among the cell lines included here are the K–562 human erythroleukemia, the YAC–1 mouse lymphoma, and the HL– 60 human leukemia lines; and liver cancer cell line.

- In contrast, cell lines of the skin and body cavity lining (epithelial) and of connective tissue, blood vessel, and lymph tissue (mesenchymal) seem to require a higher concentration of IP$_6$ in order to induce a notable effect.

In 1993, Dr Babich and colleagues used cancerous connective tissue cells (BALB/c mouse 3T3 fibroblasts) to compare the effects exerted by several nutrients that have cancer-preventing properties. Their study showed that IP$_6$ exerted a moderate degree of cell toxicity; in other words, it did not kill the cells. As disappointing it may have been to the investigators, Dr Babich's findings did not surprise us. Having carried out extensive experiments in my lab with human cancer cell lines *in vitro*, we also found IP$_6$ to have a low level of cytotoxicity as I alluded to before. It appears that IP$_6$ does not kill cells within the therapeutic dose range we used (although using a much higher dose some scientists have shown evidence of cell death), regardless of whether they are cancerous or healthy. On the other end of the spectrum, there are anti-cancer drugs that kill cells indiscriminately – making no distinction between normal cells and those that are cancerous. Do we really want them?! In contrast, within a dose range, IP₆ normalizes cancerous cells and stops them from growing aberrantly.

Research by us (Shamsuddin, Ullah & Chakravarthy, 1989; Vucenik *et al* 1993) and others (Estenson & Wattenberg, 1993) has proven that inositol by itself is also modestly effective against cancer but *only* *in vivo*; however, when it is added to IP₆, a synergistic effect appears, again only *in vivo* [it's already there in the culture media]. This means that the combination of IP₆+ inositol is far more effective against cancers than either substance administered by them. To conclude, the accumulated body of data from scientists around the globe reporting on a plurality of cancers indeed confirms that **IP₆+inositol are broad spectrum anticancer agents,** further evidence of which is presented below:

Skin Cancer

Professor Takatoshi Ishikawa and colleagues from the University of Tokyo (Ishikawa *et al* 1999) and Gupta *et al* (2003) from Lucknow, India have demonstrated that IP$_6$ inhibits experimental skin tumors, and studies at Professor David McFadden's lab have shown its efficacy against melanoma (Rizvi *et al* 2006 and Schneider *et al* 2009). Research using skin cancer cells by Huang and colleagues provides support for a theory of the underlying biochemical mechanisms whereby IP$_6$ stops or prevents cancer. Earlier, I discussed how IP$_6$ and its family of associated inositol phosphates are involved in a system of messenger cells – a system known as a signal transduction pathway. Such pathways can be activated by the presence of tumor promoters.

In the presence of an enzyme called phosphatidyl inositol-3 kinase (PI–3 kinase), a tumor promoter activates a specific protein known as protein 1 (AP–1). AP-1 makes a vital contribution to the growth of a tumor. It has been discovered that IP$_6$ has structural similarity with a substance known to be a strong inhibitor of the enzyme PI–3 kinase. This implies that IP$_6$ can inhibit (or interfere with) the activity of this enzyme and, by extension block the development of a tumor. Whereas anticancer drugs may also be designed to block the activity of PI–3 kinase, the problem remains that they are toxic. This drawback is eliminated with IP_6, which, as I mentioned several times, perhaps *ad nauseam*, is a non-toxic substance. A further significant finding of this study is that IP_6 can also directly target PI–3 kinase.

Breast Cancer

Estrogen is a hormone believed to be of great significance in the genesis and treatment of breast cancer. Some breast cancers show a growth response when specific hormones are present. In order for a tumor to respond to a certain hormone, it must have a receptor that is specific to that hormone – much like a docking station. Breast cancers are commonly tested for the presence (or absence) of estrogen or progesterone receptors (ER or PR). For instance, MCF–7 breast cancer cells are estrogen receptor-positive i.e., estrogen will bind to these receptors. In contrast, MDA MB-231 breast cancer cells are receptor-negative. Captivatingly, IP_6 has been shown to be equally successful in curtailing the growth of *both* of these cell lines. The following figure shows the pictures from such an experiment. Each of the dark blue dots represents an individual colony of cancer cells. Note that with increasing concentrations of IP₆, there is decreasing number of colonies, irrespective of the estrogen receptor status.

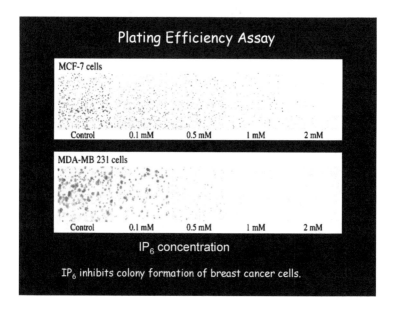

Figure 6-2: Increasing concentration of IP₆ results in decrea-sed number of colonies (dark spots) irrespective of whether the cells are estrogen-receptor-positive (MCF-7 upper panel) or estrogen-receptor-negative (MDA-MB 237 lower panel)

Prostate Cancer

Conventional approaches dictate that a breast tumor that is estrogen-positive cannot be treated the same way as one that is estrogen-negative. Similarly, PC-3 cells from prostate carcinoma require the presence of testosterone for their development (i.e., they are testosterone-dependent). In fashion, similar to the way breast cancer is handled, prostate cancer can be also treated by cutting off its source of hormones – for instance, by surgically removing the testes (orchiectomy), or by applying chemicals which eliminate the male hormones.

Dr. Guang-Yu Yang and I reported back in 1995 that as in other cancer cell lines, IP_6 not only inhibits the PC-3 prostate cancer cells, but also induces their differentiation. Subsequent extensive and ongoing investigation by Professor Rajesh Agarwal of the University of Colorado, Denver, USA on the effectiveness of IP_6 in prostate cancer is extremely encouraging.

Androgen-independent prostate cancers are harder to treat. Dr. Jean-Simon. Diallo *et al* from Centre de recherche du Centre hospitalier de l'Université de Montréal (CR-CHUM) and Institut du cancer de Montréal, report in the October 2008 issue of the *British Journal of Cancer*, that there is "[E]enhanced killing of androgen-independent prostate cancer cells when IP_6 is combined with proteasome inhibitors".

IP$_6$ Fights Rhabdomyosarcoma: A Malignant Childhood Cancer

Rhabdomyosarcomas are highly aggressive cancers of muscle; they consist of cells that appear similar to primitive skeletal muscle-forming cells. In children and in young adults, these tumors are the most prevalent soft tissue sarcomas; typically, they appear before a person turns 20. Due to their aggressive nature, these cancers are generally treated by combining radiation and chemotherapy with surgical approaches; however, in circumstances where the cancer has already spread (i.e. produced metastases), these conventional forms of therapy remain largely ineffective – the cancer usually fails to respond. There is therefore a dire need for new therapeutic approaches to fight against these cancers, as in all the rest.

Earlier, I addressed how IP$_6$ can spark a differentiation (maturation) process in human colon, prostate, and breast cancer cells. Given that rhabdomyosarcoma cells are also immature (or so-called "primitive"), my colleague Dr. Ivana Vucenik, and Dr. Thea Kalebic at the US National Cancer Institute tested whether IP$_6$ could prompt this particular

The first studies to evaluate IP_6's effects on a human rhabdomyosarcoma cell culture were performed in Petri dishes in the laboratory. Specifically, for five days we proceeded to expose RD cancer cells to various concentrations of IP_6; this was done on an uninterrupted (i.e., continuous) basis. In addition, other RD cells were also exposed to various concentrations of IP_6, but merely for periods of 6, 12, 24, or 72 hours – thereafter, the exposure to IP_6 was discontinued, and the cells were allowed to continue to grow "on their own" so to speak. The entire treatment sequence was then repeated every other day. In yet another experimental approach, additional RD cancer cells were treated with IP_6 for three days, then left on their own devices for three days (i.e., without any further addition of IP_6), then once again treated with IP_6 for another three days.

- RD cells treated continuously over a seven-day stretch with IP_6 indicated that the growth of the human rhabdomyosarcoma cell line was suppressed *in vitro* in a dose-dependent manner (i.e., increasingly higher doses suppressed growth to an additional extent);

- RD cells treated with IP_6 every second day (for 6, 12, or 24 hours) showed a response similar to the reactions noted for the RD cells treated for five days.

- Following are the results for the RD cells treated for three days with IP_6, then left untreated for three days, and then additionally treated with IP_6 for a further three days: Once IP_6 treatment had been discontinued after three days, we noted the RD cells resumed their growth; however, growth rates remained below those seen among the cells never exposed to IP_6. Once the cells were then re-exposed to IP_6, we noted a further decrease in their growth rates. Of note is the observation that the RD cells used in the experiment failed to develop a resistance to IP_6; i.e., they continued to show a reaction to IP_6's growth-reducing effect – even when exposed to IP_6 for a second time. This is significant, because in many conventional approaches to cancer treatment, the cancer cells become resistant to a drug's effects. In this instance, this did *not* happen with IP_6! Furthermore, we also considered it important that the RD cells failed to grow to any significant extent in a culture dish after they had been treated with IP_6. In contrast, when cultured in dishes, healthy and aggressive cancer cells tend to form cell colonies. Such colonies will typically grow to such an extent that they fill up the entire dish wall-to-wall with cancer cells. Such rapid growth can lead to the cells piling up on top of each other, and the cells often do not cease to grow until they have completely exhausted their entire nutrient supply contained in the culture medium. In our experiments, we found that the RD cells' capacity for building colonies was reduced once we added increasing amounts of IP₆ to the culture medium.

After exposing cancerous RD cells to IP₆, we saw some highly conspicuous morphological changes (i.e., altered shapes). Typically, untreated RD cancer cells are small and spindle-shaped. They also tend to attach themselves to the bottom of the culture dish, where they form patchy patterns; one normally does not see any evidence of skeletal muscle differentiation (maturation). We noted a change in the appearance of the cells given a second or a third three-day treatment of IP₆. These cells showed clear signs of differentiation, which is normal for *non*-cancerous cells. Specifically, the treated cells grew larger and produced higher levels of the so-called muscle-specific actin (a protein found explicitly in normal, differentiated skeletal muscle cells). RD cancer cells cannot produce muscle-specific actin. In here too, we noted a proclivity of the RD cells exposed to IP$_6$ to take on normal shapes and functions; this tendency remained constant - even in view of a minimum of 3 – 4 passages of cells into a new culture medium.

We were also interested in seeing IP$_6$'s potential effects on human cancer cells *in vivo* (i.e., in a live person or animal). Typically, human cancer cells are introduced into an animal and then the animal is treated with a specific anticancer. This procedure is performed before one actually administers anticancer substances to humans who have cancer. In our experiment, we used mice that lacked the thymus gland (these are so-called athymic 'nude' mice, nude because they are hairless) to study the impact IP$_6$ would have on the RD cells' tumor-forming capacity. The thymus is a vital constituent of our immune system. Having access to animals without a thymus allowed us to introduce (transplant) human tumor cells into the mice, giving us the opportunity to evaluate how effective certain anticancer agents are in fighting this *human* cancer in the study animals.

We proceeded to inject each mouse with live human RD cells. Injections were made under the animals' skins in the lower back region. Following this procedure, we injected IP_6 around the developing tumors, administering a dose of 40 mg of IP_6 per kilogram of body weight. For comparative purposes, in a 70-kg human this amount would roughly equal 2800 mg (or 2.8 g) of IP_6. This treatment was initiated two days after the mice had been injected with the tumor cells. We continued to treat the mice in this fashion every second day, three times per week – the procedure was continued either for two weeks (in "Experiment 1") or for five weeks (in "Experiment 2"). Control animals were also injected with tumor cells, but they did not receive any IP_6. We cared for all the mice in accordance with institutional guidelines that have been laid out to ensure experimental animals are treated humanely, as we have so done in *all* of the experiments we conducted. Twice a week, we monitored the mice for tumor growth; we also checked them for other potential growth deformities.

Tumors developed in all the control animals (i.e., the mice that had not been given IP_6). In the animals treated with IP_6, we could see a considerable reduction in tumor growth; in fact, treatment with IP_6 was associated not only with a lower incidence of tumors, but the tumors were also much smaller. The tumors appeared in 40% of the animals from "Experiment 1" as well as in 20% of the mice from "Experiment 2". In those instances, where tumors did appear in animals treated with IP₆, we found that they were 25 - 49 times smaller than the tumors in the control animals! We also found that the IP₆- treated animals that developed tumors did so 25 days 25 days after RD cells injection. In contrast, in the control animals, tumors were developing after 10 days.

In regards to IP₆'s suppressive effect on RD cell growth, our *in vivo* studies with athymic mice corroborated the earlier results achieved *in vitro* (i.e., in cell culture experiments). I already drew your attention to the fact that following two weeks of treatment the mice given IP₆ developed tumors that were 25 times smaller than the tumors we found in the control animals (Experiment 1). In the second experiment (Experiment 2) we treated mice with IP₆ for a period of 4 weeks. This more drawn-out study yielded a 49-fold reduction in tumor size ($p=0.001$)! In a follow-up analysis using a microscope, we found no evidence of necrosis (a form of cell death where cells break open and release their contents) among these tumor cells. This finding serves to confirm what we had gleaned from all our previous experiments, namely that IP$_6$ does not kill tumor cells. This might be a good way to halt cancer cells. In some instances, radiation treatments and chemotherapeutic drugs prompt tumor cells to undergo necrosis very quickly, thereby littering a patient's body with large quantities of toxic tumor debris and dead cancer cells. But IP$_6$, which is non-toxic manages to stall the growth of cancer cells and suppress tumor growth by a factor of 29 - 49!

This marked and statistically significant reduction in tumor growth (p=0.008 to 0.001) was consistent over two independent studies. The tumors we found in IP$_6$-treated and in untreated mice looked the same; however, the tumors of the treated group showed a lower mitotic rate. In other words, the tumor cells in the IP$_6$-treated mice were dividing and multiplying at a slower pace. This once again underscores how effectively IP$_6$ inhibits the growth of tumors, and how it stimulates human RD cells to undergo maturation process. Given the dramatic effects we found in these studies (on live animals), we surmise that IP$_6$ is also able to curb the growth of human rhabdomyosarcomas.

A further finding to come out of these experiments is that the cancer cells do not become resistant to IP_6 at least not in this model. In summary, all of our studies point to IP_6 having a great potential in fighting rhabdomyosarcoma, as well as other related tumors.

IP_6 in Liver Cancer

Liver cancer (also known as hepatocellular carcinoma) is common in areas where the hepatitis B virus is widespread (such as in China). North America's incidence of liver cancer ranges between 3 - 7 cases per 100,000 people; however, the liver cancer found here is predominantly associated with liver cirrhosis - caused by alcohol, excessive iron, and prompted by other toxins. Whatever its cause, liver cancer is a malignant disease with only a very minimal chance for a positive outcome - death often occurs within half a year of the cancer's diagnosis. While numerous therapeutic approaches have been suggested, their effectiveness remains tentative.

In the summer of 1997, I was visited by Dr. Zhenshu Zhang from the Nanfang Hospital of the First PLA Medical College in Guangzhou, China. He did not approach me with any specific project, but casually educated me about China's endeavors to treat human liver cancer by injecting alcohol directly into tumors. At that time, I took an interest on IP_6's potential to treat liver cancer. We decided to conduct a pilot study to evaluate whether IP_6 might be able to suppress the generation and development of cancer cells in humans. Because this study was likely to be very costly – both in financial terms, as well as in view of its heavy exploitation of research animals – we decided to test first whether human cancer cells would show any response at all to IP_6. Our reasoning for taking this approach was that if human cancer cells were to be *un*responsive to IP_6 in an *in vitro* environment (i.e., in a lab setting), then we could forgo further experimental studies involving research animals. Adopting this approach, we proceeded to harvest human liver cancer cells (HepG2) and cultivated them in the lab, applying IP_6 to some of the cells, but not to others (control - without IP_6 treatment).

We discovered that treatment with IP_6 suppressed the growth of these human cancer cells. In addition, we found that the growth inhibition response was dose-dependent. In fact, the cancer cells were highly responsive to IP_6's cancer-fighting powers - some of the cancerous cells even ceased to grow entirely when given sufficient IP_6.

These exciting results begged follow-up experiment that entailed the injection of human liver
cancer cells into nude mice. 71% of the mice that
had not received any IP$_6$ prior to being exposed to
the cancer cells developed large tumors. In contrast, the mice that had received HepG2 cells treated *in vitro* with IP$_6$ 48 hours prior to inoculation
remained tumor-free. Thus, exposure to IP$_6$ somehow brought the cancerous tumor cells' aberrant
and rampant growth to a halt and prevented them
from growing into a tumor. In the other part of the
experiment, even in the mice that did establish
tumors, a treatment with IP$_6$ still produced favorable outcomes: Once the tumors in these animals
reached 8 - 10 mm in diameter (in a human, this
would correspond to a tumor the size of a basket-
ball), we injected them with IP$_6$ for 12 days in a
row. The IP$_6$-treated mice then showed a 3.4-fold
reduction in tumor weights (compared to the control animals that went without IP$_6$). The 'star of the
show' was animal number 11 whose tumor had
completely regressed during a mere 1 week period
while that in a control animal grew 2-3 folds
within that period (*Anticancer Research* volume
18: pages 4091-4096, 1998).

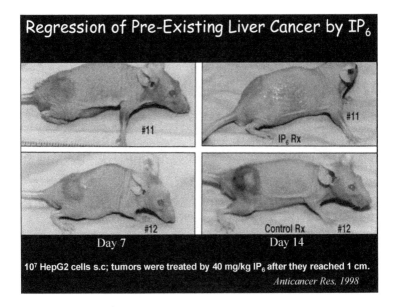

Figure 6-3: The tumor in mouse #11 has totally regressed in a week during the period its sibling #12 has 2-3-fold larger tumor.

What intrigued us most about these experimental findings was the fact that a single IP₆ treatment somehow rendered the cancerous cells completely powerless – they could no longer produce tumors. In contrast, those cells left untreated did produce tumors in the mice. IP₆'s profound effect on preexisting liver cancer cells was even more noteworthy: Cancerous liver cells exposed directly to IP₆ responded to the treatment with growth regression. The study thereby proves that IP₆ can be applied successfully to treat very malignant hepatocellular carcinoma.

Monitoring the Efficacy of IP$_6$ Treatment by Tumor Marker

We also asked the question: Would IP$_6$ decrease the tumor marker levels used to monitor the progression of the cancer and/or efficacy of treatment in addition to decreasing the rate of cell proliferation and tumor formation [This is an extension of the question we asked with colon cancer model using Gal-GalNAc as the surrogate marker]? In our earlier experiments, we have found that IP$_6$ causes a concomitant differentiation of cancer cells to normal appearing ones along with a reduction in cell proliferation. These were seen as increased cytokeratin expression in HT-29 human colon cancer cells, lactalbumin in breast cancer cells etc. More in line with the current day practice, the tumor marker α-fetoprotein (AFP) is in standard use to monitor liver cancer - increased amount of it in the blood is a sign of increased tumor load, and *vice versa*. HepG2 cells, as in liver cancer in a patient produce AFP. We thus tested for the expression of AFP in the culture media and in HepG2 cells following IP$_6$ treatment in the Petri dishes in the laboratory. We found that concurrent to cancer cell inhibition; there was a rather dramatic decrease in AFP production. Note in Table 6-1 that following 1 mM IP_6 treatment, there was a virtual shutdown of AFP production. Thus, the efficacy of IP_6+inositol treatment can be monitored by routine periodic follow-up of tumor markers.

Table 6-1: Effect of IP_6 Treatment on α Fetoprotein (AFP) Secretion in HepG2 Cells

Treatment	AFP in Media ng/mL	AFP in Cells pg/Cell
0 IP_6 (Control)	$1,3790 \pm 65.7$	27.6 ± 1.3
0.5 mM IP_6	63.0 ± 24.0	5.3 ± 2.0
1.0 mM IP_6	1.9 ± 0.2	0.3 ± 0.0

Difference between control v Treatment groups is significant at $p<0.0001$.

On the topic of monitoring cancer patients following initial treatment, as you had read in Chapter 1 and earlier in this chapter, the tumor marker Gal-GalNAc is expressed in patients with various cancers making it a common marker for their screening. Drs. Kosaku Sakamoto from Japan and Guang-yu Yang from Shenyang, China while working in my laboratory independently and at different times had shown that IP_6 treatment of human colon cancer cells decrease and may even completely shut-off Gal-GalNAc production. Thus, individuals who are screen positive and are treated or taking prophylactic IP_6+inositol could be easily monitored by repeat screening test for Gal-Gal-NAc.

Melanoma, Glioblastoma etc.

As if the preceding is not sufficient, the broad-spectrum anticancer action of IP_6±Inositol has been further proven by the demonstration of growth inhibition of skin cancer melanoma (Schneider *et al* 2009), brain tumor glioblastoma (Karmakar *et al* 2007), oral cavity squamous cell carcinoma (Janus *et al* 2007) etc. *in vitro*.

CHAPTER 7

CLINICAL STUDIES OF HUMAN CANCER TREATMENT

What Should Be The Properties Of Good Anticancer Agents?

A good anticancer agent needs to be selective: it should only affect malignant cells and spare normal cells and tissues. This property was shown for IP_6. When the fresh $CD34^+$ cells from bone marrow was treated with different doses of IP_6, an inhibition of growth was observed that was specific to leukemic progenitors from chronic myelogenous leukemia patients, but no cytotoxic or cytostatic effect was observed on normal bone marrow progenitor cells under the same conditions. In another type of experiments, IP_6 inhibited the colony formation of Kaposi Sarcoma cell lines, KS Y-1 (AIDS-related KS cell line) and KS SLK (Iatrogenic KS) and CCRF-CEM (human adult T lymphoma) cells in a dose-dependent manner; however, in striking contrast to the anticancer drug Taxol used as a control, IP_6 did not affect the ability of normal cells (peripheral blood mononuclear cells and colony-forming T cells) to form colonies in a semisolid methylcellulose medium.

Malignant and normal cells are known to have different metabolisms, growth rate, expression of receptors, etc., but the mechanism for this different selectivity of IP_6 for normal and malignant cells needs to be further investigated. Current cancer treatment recognizes the power of combination therapy to increase efficacy – we need all the help we can get, from anywhere! It would be self-defeating to have a closed-mind.

Another important aspect of cancer treatment is overcoming acquired drug resistance. Our studies demonstrate that *in vitro*, IP$_6$ acts synergistically with doxorubicin and tamoxifen, being particularly effective against estrogen receptor–negative and doxorubicin-resistant tumor cell lines, both conditions that are challenging to treat (Tantivejkul *et al* 2003 a). These data are particularly important as tamoxifen is usually given as a chemopreventive agent in the post-treatment period and doxorubicin has enormous cardiotoxicity and its use is associated with doxorubicin resistance. Emerging clinical data (please see below) support that IP$_6$+inositol when used in combination with standard chemotherapeutic agents augment the latter's ability to control tumor growth.

Clinical Studies of IP$_6$ & Inositol

While the laboratory data have shown consistent and reproducible anti-cancer and other health benefits of IP$_6$+Inositol since the late 1980's and has been available as a dietary supplement beginning 1998, only recently it has been getting the attention of academic physicians, numerous self-reporting by the patients notwithstanding. And here they are:

IP₆ (with β-Glucan)

Dr. Alan Weitberg from the Department of Medicine at Roger Williams Medical Center, Providence, Rhode Island and Boston University School of Medicine, Boston, Massachusetts reports in *Journal of Experimental and Clinical Cancer Research* (2008) the results of a phase I/II clinical trial of β-(1,3)/(1,6) D-glucan + IP₆ in the treatment of patients with advanced malignancies receiving chemotherapy. β-Glucan is a long chain polymer of glucose derived from the fungal cell wall; it has been shown to have a number of immunomodulatory properties as well as effects on hematopoiesis and as a radiation protectant.

Twenty patients with advanced malignancies receiving chemotherapy were given a β-glucan preparation plus IP₆ and monitored for tolerability and effect on hematopoiesis. Dr. Weitberg reports that β-glucan + IP₆ is well-tolerated in cancer patients receiving chemotherapy and may have a beneficial effect on hematopoiesis in these patients, especially in those with chronic lymphocytic leukemia and lymphoma. However, owing to the mixture of β-glucan with IP₆, both seeming to have similar effect it was not clear from the paper as to how much of the reported results can be attributed to either IP$_6$ or β-glucan or the combination thereof. Attempts to obtain clarification from Dr. Weitberg were unsuccessful.

Myo-Inositol

Myo-Inositol has been considered to be safe and essential enough to be included not only as a member of B-vitamin family, but is a necessary component of baby formulas as well as growth media for keeping cell in the lab alive (culturing). It has already been in therapeutic use, in large dosage (up to 12 g/day) for certain neuropsychiatric disorders (Levine 1997); more on it later.

From the British Columbia Cancer Agency, Vancouver, Canada Dr. Stephen Lam and colleagues from the Universities of British Columbia and Minnesota, and the US National Cancer Institute in Bethesda, Maryland report on a Phase I, open-label, multiple dose, dose-escalation clinical study to assess the safety, tolerability, maximum tolerated dose, and potential chemopreventive effect of *myo*-inositol in smokers with bronchial dysplasia - precursor of lung cancer. A dose escalation study ranging from 12 to 30 g/day of *myo*-inositol for a month was first conducted in 16 subjects to determine the maximum tolerated dose. Ten new subjects were then enrolled to take the maximum tolerated dose for 3 months. The researchers also investigated the potential chemopreventive effect of *myo*-inositol by repeat auto-fluorescence bronchoscopy and biopsy. The maximum tolerated dose was found to be 18 g/day. Side effects, when present, were mild and mainly gastrointestinal in nature. A significant increase in the rate of regression of preexisting dysplastic lesions was observed (91% versus 48%; $P = 0.014$). A **statistically significant reduction in the systolic and diastolic blood pressures** by an average of 10 mm Hg was observed after taking 18 g/d of *myo*-inositol for a month or more.

Dr. Adam Gutafson and colleagues at the Boston University Medical Center, University of Utah in Salt Lake City, Vanderbilt-Ingram Comprehensive Cancer Center in Nashville TN, and the National Cancer Institute in Bethesda, MD in USA and British Columbia Cancer Agency in Vancouver, Canada report in the 7 April 2010 issue of *Science Translational Medicine* (2:26ra25) a significant increase in the genomic signature of phosphatidylinositol 3-kinase (PI3K) pathway activation in the cytologically normal bronchial cells of smokers with lung cancer and precancerous lesions; *myo*-

inositol decreased the PI3 kinase activity in the airway of high-risk smokers with a concomitant significant regression of precancerous dysplasia. The results were exciting enough to deserve coverage by the NBC Nightly News in USA on 7 April 2010. http://www.msnbc.msn.com/id/3032619/#36239305

IP₆+Inositol and Colorectal Cancer

At the 17th Annual Meeting of the European Association for Cancer Research in Grenada, Spain (8-11 June, 2002) Professor Nikica Družijanić from the Clinical Hospital Split in Split, Croatia presented the very first study of the use of IP₆+ Inositol in cancer patients. He reported (*Revista de Oncología* volume 4, Supplement 1, Pages 1-179, Abstract #480) the results of a pilot study on six patients (age 51-70 years) with advanced colorectal cancer (Dukes C and D) receiving standard chemotherapy and IP₆+Inositol.

"Chemotherapy related side effects (nausea, vomiting, alopecia, diarrhea, paresthesis, etc.) were minimal and patients were able to perform their daily activities."

One patient with liver metastasis abstained from chemotherapy after first treatment; and she was being treated with IP$_6$+Inositol (12 capsules per day) alone. "…ultrasound and abdominal CT 14 months postoperatively have shown significantly reduced tumor growth rate and her liver tests are slightly increased." reported Prof. Družijanić.

A 2-day long special IP$_6$+Inositol Symposium "IP$_6$ and Inositol in Cell Signaling: *From Laboratory to Clinic*" was held as part of the 7th International Conference of Anticancer Research in Corfu, Greece, October 25-30, 2004. More than 20 eminent scientists from North America, Europe, Africa and Asia presented papers on various aspects of research on inositol phosphates and inositol, as the title states, from basic science research in the laboratory to clinical studies with patients, and everything in between. Data from four clinical studies, 2 each from Croatia and Japan were presented. Professor Nikica Družijanić and his colleagues at the Clinical Hospital, Split, Croatia reported an enhanced anticancer activity without compromising the patient's quality of life in a pilot clinical trial involving 22 patients with advanced colorectal cancer (Duke's B2, C and D) with multiple liver and lung metastasis. The age range was 42-71 years. During the chemo- and radiotherapy the patients were monitored with CBC (complete blood count) with differentials, creatinine, electrolytes, various enzyme markers and the tumor markers CEA and CA 19-9.

The patients were surgically operated and subjected to adjuvant polychemotherapy according to the Mayo protocol. IP₆+Inositol were given as an adjuvant to chemotherapy during and after the chemotherapy for a one year period. A reduced tumor growth rate was noticed overall, and in some cases a regression of lesions was noted. Additionally, when IP₆+Inositol was given in combination with chemotherapy, side effects of chemotherapy, such as drop in leukocyte and platelet counts, nausea, vomiting, alopecia, were diminished and patients were able to perform their daily activities.

"All patients treated with adjuvant polychemotherapy...and IP6+ inositol had significantly reduced chemotherapy-related side-effects (drop in leukocytes and platelet counts, nausea, vomiting, fever, diarrhea and alopecia). All of the laboratory parameters during therapy were within normal range. Thus, in contrast to standard chemotherapy-alone regimen wherein we are often forced to stop the chemo owing to severe side-effects it was never necessary to interrupt the chemotherapy in patients on adjuvant inositol +

IP6." (Anticancer Research volume 24, No. 5D, September-October, 2004 page 3474, paper #125).

Figure 7-1 shows the abdominal CT scan of a 63 years old man with inoperable Stage IV colorectal cancer with metastases in liver and lungs, before and 4 months after initiation of IP₆+Inositol treatment.

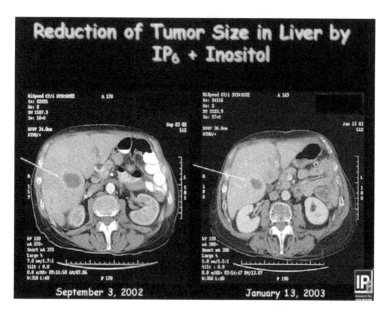

Figure 7-1: The arrows point to the metastatic liver cancer before (left panel) and 4 months after IP₆+Inositol treatment.

IP₆+Inositol and Breast Cancer

At the same meeting in Corfu, Greece, Drs. Kosa-ku Sakamoto and Yoshihiko Suzuki from Sakamo-to Clinic of Gastroenterology and Takasaki National Hospital, Gunma, Japan presented a case of a 79 years old patient with metastatic breast cancer treated with IP₆+Inositol (Paper #438). The patient had developed pleural effusion secondary to the metastases at which time she was started on IP₆+Inositol in April 2002. "Four months later, the tumor markers had dropped to a normal level. An additional 2 months later, the pleural effusion decreased in volume. However, it began to increase in volume in May 2003. The tumor markers also increased continuously thereafter, reaching 35- to 40- fold higher than normal level in July 2004. While the signs of metastatic disease show progression, her general condition is not impaired and quality of life status remains favorable." Drs. Sakamoto & Suzuki opine "[T]the reason for the patient's favorable condition, in spite of a large burden of the relapsed tumor mass, may be partly attributed to the fact that she has taken IP6 + Inositol every day for more than two years." They conclude "[I]in combination with an oral intake of chemotherapeutic agents (anti-estrogen agent and tegafur-uracil mixture), IP6 + Inositol may contribute to improved quality of life and prolonged survival of patients with metastatic recurrence of breast cancer."

In here, Prof. Družijanić also presented a pilot study on 4 patients with ductal invasive breast cancer in stage II and IIIa, all treated with chemotherapy and radiotherapy, and IP₆+Inositol (Paper #126). He too reports that the patients' quality of life was superior and the side-effects secondary to chemo- and radiation-therapy were minimal.

More recently, in 2010 Prof. Družijanić and his colleague published a paper in the *Journal of Experimental and Clinical Cancer Research* describing the results of a prospective randomized pilot clinical study of 14 breast cancer patients treated with IP₆+Inositol. Patients receiving chemotherapy, along with IP₆+Inositol did not have drop in leukocyte and platelet counts as opposed to controls. Patients who took IP₆+Inositol had significantly better quality of life (statistically significant at $p=0.05$) and functional status (statistically highly significant at $p=0.0003$) and were able to perform their daily activities.

All of the patients enrolled in the study had filled the questionnaires QLQ-30 and QLQ-BR23 from

European organization for testing the treatment of cancer (EORTC). The questions in questionnaire were divided into the functional and symptomatic scales. The Functional scale contains questions about the physical, emotional, cognitive, social and sexual functions. Each group has a range of responses matching from 0-100 wherein a score of 100 represents the maximum compatibility with the offered answers; and 0 represents the complete lack of compatibility.

Table 7-1:   Quality of Life Assessment

Quality of Life		
Patients	**Mean ± SD**	***p* value**
Placebo Group (7)	48.43 ± 28.96	0.05
IP₆ + Inositol Group (7)	78.33 ± 21.60	

Based on patients' on personal assessment

Table 7-2:   Functional Status Assessment

Functional Status		
Patients	**Mean ± SD**	***p* value**
Placebo Group	56.29 ± 15.32	0.0003
IP₆ + Inositol Group	87.94 ± 6.94	

Based on patients' on personal assessment

The Symptomatic scale contains questions about side-effects of treatment, such as the general bad condition, nausea, vomiting, diarrhea, constipation, pain, insomnia, and loss of appetite, loss of body weight, hair loss, increase in body temperature and the operating complications of treatment. Replies from symptomatic scale are evaluated with the scale from 0-100, where 100 represents maximal positive personal experience with total quality of life; and 0 represent the most negative personal experience of the quality of life.

Patients' self-assessments of chemotherapy-induced symptoms are presented in the following Table 7-3.

Table 7-3:   Chemotherapy Side-Effects: Symptomatic

Clinical Symptoms of Side-Effects		
Patients	Mean ± SD	*p* value
Placebo Group	33.81 ± 18.12	0.04
IP₆+Inositol Group	13.51 ± 9.98	

Based on patients' on personal assessment

While the patient self-reporting is subjective, it is imperative that objective evidence in the form of changes on white blood cells (WBC), platelets counts and other laboratory parameters are evaluated. As almost all, if not all patients undergoing chemotherapy and/or radiation treatment are painfully aware of, decrease in these parameters result in lowered immunity (WBC) with resultant increased risk of infection and frequent and serious bleeding (platelets). Table 7-4 presents the data on the WBC and platelets before and after treatment with and without IP₆+Inositol.

Table 7-4: Chemotherapy Side-Effects On Blood Cell Counts

Blood Cell		Placebo Mean ± SD	IP₆ + Inositol Mean ± SD
WBC (x10⁹/L)	Before Rx	7.53 ± 1.50	6.66 ± 0.96
	After Rx	4.36 ± 1.80	6.92 ± 2.12
	p value	0.01	0.75
Platelets (x10⁹/L)	Before Rx	272.71 ± 114.86	229.57 ± 31.81
	After Rx	205.00 ± 90.56	231.86 ± 47.33
	p value	0.05	0.92

Note that the decrease in WBC counts in placebo group is statistically significant whereas those in IP₆+Inositol treated group are not; there was no decrease in platelet counts with IP₆+Inositol.

The authors concluded "IP₆ + Inositol as an adjunctive therapy is valuable help in ameliorating the side effects and preserving quality of life among the patients treated with chemotherapy."

IP₆+Inositol and Lung Cancer

From Japan Dr. Kosaku Sakamoto also presented in Corfu, Greece, a case-report of long-term survival of a patient with non-small cell carcinoma of the lung (Paper # 439). A 59-years old female with a smoking history of 30 years was diagnosed with adenocarcinoma of her left lung (T2N3M0, Stage IIIB) at the age of 49. She was undergoing chemo-radiotherapy which was discontinued in midcourse owing to intractable side-effects. She was started on IP₆+Inositol 8 months following cessation of standard therapy. Of particular note is that the *patient has not been taking any other medications during this period*.

Four years and 4 months hence, she has been enjoying a "completely healthy life without any signs of relapse. Periodic check-up of her chest and abdomen by computed tomography (CT) and, recently, by multi-detector CT, revealed no evidence of tumor regression...Serum CEA level drastically decreased to normal when the CRT [chemo-radiotherapy] was terminated, and continues to be normal." Himself having conducted some elegant experimental work on IP₆ and Inositol in the early 1990's, Dr. Sakamoto as a clinician concludes "[N]neither IP6 nor inositol have [*sic*] any adverse effect on humans, which is most important for a candidate therapeutic agent, and more importantly for long-term use as a preventive agent against cancer."

CHAPTER 8

MECHANISMS OF ACTION OF IP₆ & INOSITOL

It seems that classification or grouping people or actions are almost a constant phenomenon in life. People are grouped according to different identifiable characteristics such as race, ethnicity, religion, political affiliation etc. And so are many other things. There are people who are "lumpers" – groups that do not wish to divide or classify and "spli-tters," who do. IP₆ and inositol may bring about their actions in various ways; and so, I am often pressured to classify them. I am not sure that this classification is accurate, but the mechanisms may be broadly looked at as biological, cellular, mole-cular, etc. with some overlap, which makes it diffi-cult to make rigid classification. You will note that immunity plays a very important role in cancer for-mation and control, as well as in many other disea-ses; an entire chapter is dedicated to that. For now, let's look at some of the ways how IP₆ and inositol act.

Cell Survival, Proliferation and Differentiation

IP₆ and inositol affect all the stages in a cell's life: survival (or death), cell division (or proliferation) and cell differentiation. In the body, most cells are associated with others forming a society or tissue wherein they need mechanical strength for which not only they interact with each other, but also are interdependent. The extracellular matrix for exam-ple provides the epithelial cells with this mechani-cal support.

Apoptosis

It has been estimated that in every second approximately a million cells die in our body, mostly through pre-programmed death. In the skin and the gut lumen, the dead cells simply slough off, or are quickly swallowed up by healthy neighbors or scavenger cells – the macrophages. This process of cell death is also called apoptosis, as opposed to necrosis wherein cells die as a result of injury. How do the 'professional' scavenger cells know when and where to find the apoptotic cells so that they can be quickly removed? Dr. Michael R. Elliott and his colleagues at University of Virginia, Charlottesville and University of North Carolina, Chapel Hill show that the apoptotic cells send at least one group of 'find me' signals to the macrophages; the molecules are ATP and UTP (*Nature* 461: 282, 10 Sept 2009).

Since the standard chemotherapeutic agents work by killing cells, I was not much interested in looking at cell-killing by IP₆; one could say that I almost had an aversion towards that! Thus, we set our experiments to rather not see apoptosis! Instead we looked for decreased cell proliferation and differentiation which we will discuss later in this chapter. Others who followed our work were more interested in apoptosis; subsequently they used either different cell lines and/or higher concentrations of IP_6 and reported apoptosis.

At concentrations up to 2-5 mM, IP_6 inhibits cell proliferation of cancer cell lines with concomitant induced differentiation, but without a substantial increase in cell death in most cell lines. However, at higher dosage, or on prolonged treatment it induces apoptosis or programmed cell death. HeLa cells on the other hand appear to be more sensitive, undergoing apoptosis at IP_6 concentrations where very little apoptosis was observed in other cell lines. The first such report of apoptosis by IP_6 came from Prof. Masato Hirata's lab in Fukuoka, Japan. They treated uterine cancer HeLa[1] cells with IP_6 which induced apoptosis. Induction of apoptosis by IP_6 was examined in two ways: inhibition of cell survival signaling and direct induction of apoptosis. Treatment of HeLa cells with tumor necrosis factor (TNF) or insulin stimulated the Akt-nuclear factor κB (NFκB) pathway, a cell survival signal, which involves the phosphoryla-

---

[1] HeLa cells are immortalized cells from the cervical cancer of Henrietta Lacks who died of her cancer on 4 October, 1951 at the Johns Hopkins Hospital in Baltimore; she too is immortalized through her gift!

tion of Akt and IκB, nuclear translocation of NFkB and NFkB-luciferase transcription activity. IP_6 blocked all these cellular events. IP_6 itself caused mitochondrial permeabilization, followed by cytochrome c release, which later caused activation of the apoptotic machinery, caspase 9, caspase 3 and poly (ADP-ribose) polymerase. They conclude that exogenously applied IP_6 directly activates the apoptotic machinery as well as inhibits the cell survival signaling, probably by the intracellular delivery followed by a dephosphorylation.

In line with the broad-spectrum anticancer activity of IP_6, induction of apoptosis is also seen in other cancers. Prof. Rajesh Agarwal's group at the University of Colorado Health Sciences Center in Denver has been contributing significantly towards the treatment and prevention of prostate cancer. They have used advanced human prostate cancer cells DU145 to investigate the mechanisms of action of IP_6. "At higher doses and longer treatment times, IP_6 caused a marked increase in apoptosis, which was accompanied by increased levels of cleaved PARP and active caspase 3. IP_6 modulates CDKI-CDK-cyclin complex, and decreases CDK-cyclin kinase activity, possibly leading to hypophosphorylation of Rb-related proteins and an increased sequestration of E2F4. Higher doses

of IP_6 could induce apoptosis and that might involve caspases activation."

They then expanded their work on TRAMP cells
(transgenic adenocarcinoma of mouse prostate),
which reproduces the spectrum of benign latent,
aggressive and metastatic forms of human prostatic carcinoma. TRAMP-C1 cell line was treated
with IP_6 which resulted in cell death (apoptosis)
with concurrent inhibition of cell growth in a dose-
and time-dependent manner. IP_6 induced a moderate to strong (up to 14-fold over control) apoptotic
cell death. Pretreatment of cells with caspases inhibitor for 2 h followed by 2 mM IP_6 for 48 h resulted in approximately 50% reversal in IP_6-induced
apoptosis suggesting a partial involvement of caspases activation in apoptosis caused by IP_6. IP_6
also showed a 6-fold induction in caspase-3 activity compared to control, again suggesting the
involvement of caspases activation in IP_6-induced
apoptosis. Evidence was gathered that implicated
the involvement of both caspase-dependent and -
independent mechanisms in IP_6-induced apoptotic
death of TRAMP-C1 cells.

*"Our results suggest that IP6 could be a potent
dietary agent in controlling the growth of advanced PCA cells and inducing their apoptotic dea-*

th, in part, by its inhibitory effect on constitutively active NF-kappa B signaling pathway."

Further work from Prof. Agarwal's lab show that apoptosis can be induced also *in vivo*: IP_6 increases cyclin-dependent kinase inhibitors p21/Cip1 and p27/Kip1 protein levels in human prostate cancer DU145 cells lacking functional p53. IP_6-induced apoptosis occurred in a Cip/Kip-dependent manner in cell culture and xenograft. They also provided evidence that p21 and p27 have a critical role in mediating the anticancer efficacy of IP_6 both *in vitro* and *in vivo*.

While much of the work on apoptosis by IP_6 was performed in the *in vitro* cell culture system [it is much easier to induce and observe here than in animal systems], that apoptosis indeed takes place *in vivo* has been also proven. The first report comes from the laboratory of Drs. Jenab and Thompson, then at the University of Toronto, Canada. Male Fischer 344 rats were injected with colon-carcinogen and fed a basal control diet or one supplemented with either, wheat bran, or wheat bran stripped of IP_6 or wheat bran stripped of IP_6 + added IP_6 to dissect out if the results are due to IP_6. They observed that IP_6 significantly increased the rate of apoptosis in the crypts. They concluded that wheat bran, partly due to its dietary fiber and endogenous IP_6, and exogenous IP_6 when added to a low fiber diet can increase cell apoptosis and differentiation and favorably affect colon morphology of apoptosis in the crypts of colonic epithelial cells.

Gupta *et al* (2003) from the Industrial Toxicology Research Center, Lucknow, India investigated the effect of topical application of IP_6 on 7,12-dimethylbenzanthracene (DMBA)-induced carcinogenesis of mouse skin. Along with a significant inhibition of skin tumor development IP_6 induced DMBA-inhibited transglutaminase activity. DNA synthesis, as determined by ^{3}H-thymidine incorporation, was suppressed by IP_6 in a dose-dependent manner. IP_6 also inhibited thymidine kinase enzyme, which is responsible for ^{3}H-thymidine incorporation into DNA. They thus showed that topical application of IP_6 inhibits DMBA-induced mouse skin tumor development and that IP_6 exerts its tumor inhibitory effect probably by modulating proliferation, differentiation, or apoptosis. "It seems that IP_6 is an effective and potential chemopreventive agent for management of skin tumorigenesis."

Now, here is the apparent paradox: In contrast to induction of apoptosis in cancer-prone cells, IP_6 can attenuate apoptosis where apoptosis is harmful! Drs. Aljandali, Kamp and colleagues at the Northwestern University Medical School and the Veterans Administration Health Care in Chicago report that IP_6 reduces asbestos-induced apoptosis in alveolar epithelial cells in the lungs. We shall discuss more on this later in the context of oxidative damage and its modulation by IP_6.

Anoikis

One of the most dangerous weapon in cancer cells' arsenal is their ability to detach from their habitat, invade surrounding tissues and travel to distant sites to cause havoc there (metastasis). But when otherwise normal cells are removed from natural surrounding such as loss of extracellular matrix attachment to cultured epithelial cells, they undergo self-destruction or *anoikis* (derived from Greek to mean "homelessness"). Originally, it was presumed that anoikis is executed by apoptosis; but that has changed. Recent research show that blocking apoptosis does not prevent anoikis; detached cells die any way! Anoikic cells undergo a process whereby the cell digests parts of itself (autophagocytosis or autophagy). Autophagy may help the cell survive starvation, but if it runs its full course, it may cause cellular death through self-consumption. Since cancer cells have the ability to invade, naturally they escape anoikis. One may look at it in another manner and argue that anoikis prevents cancer! That remains to be seen and so is the role of IP₆, if any in anoikis. But thanks to Schafer *et al* (2009) who recently showed that oxidative stress induces anoikis and certain anti-oxidants prevent it; this would suggest that anti-oxidants may not have a beneficial effect in cancer treatment. Not only this is the first study of its kind, but it was also performed in an *in vitro* system. So, don't rush to throw your anti-oxidants away.

Cell Proliferation

Since IP₆ inhibits cell division, its effect on the cell cycle and these cell cycle regulatory proteins and their genes have been looked at. Using DU145 human prostate cancer cell line, Singh *et al* (2003, 2004) studied the cell cycle progression and apoptosis by flow cytometry. They also investigated the involvement of G_1 cell cycle regulators and their interplay and end point markers of apoptosis. A significant dose- and time-dependent growth inhibition of IP$_6$-treated cells was associated with an increase in cells in G$_1$. IP$_6$ strongly increased the expression of cyclin-dependent kinase inhibitors (CDKIs) - Cip1/p21 and Kip1/p27, without any noticeable changes in G$_1$ CDKs and cyclins, except a slight increase in cyclin D2. IP$_6$ inhibited kinase activities associated with CDK2, 4 and 6, and cyclin E and D1. Further studies showed the increased binding of Kip1/p27 and Cip1/p21 with cyclin D1 and E. In down-stream of CDKI-CDK/cyclin cascade, IP$_6$ increased hypophosphorylated levels of Rb-related proteins, pRb/p107 and pRb2/p130, and moderately decreased E2F4 but increased its binding to both pRb/p107 and pRb2/p130. At higher doses and longer treatment times, IP$_6$ caused a marked increase in apoptosis, which was accompanied by increased levels of cleaved PARP and active caspase 3. IP$_6$ modulated CDKI-CDK-cyclin complex, and decreases CDK-cyclin kinase activity, possibly leading to hypophosphorylation of Rb-related proteins and an increased sequestration of E2F4. Higher doses of IP$_6$ could induce apoptosis and that might involve caspases activation.

TRAMP-C1 cell line was treated with IP$_6$ which resulted in cell death (apoptosis) with concomitant inhibition of cell growth in a dose- and time-dependent manner (Sharma *et al* 2003). In the studies assessing whether cell growth inhibition by IP_6 is associated with an alteration in cell cycle progression, IP_6 treatment resulted in up to 92% cells in G_0-G_1 phase as compared to controls.

Wheat bran (WB) and its component IP_6 have both been shown to decrease early biomarkers of colon carcinogenesis, i.e. the PCNA labeling index of cell proliferation and certain aberrant crypt foci parameters. (Jenab & Thompson)

Differentiation

In general, cell differentiation depends on changes in gene expression resulting in synthesis and accumulation of different sets of RNA and consequently protein molecules; the latter often represent the differentiated features. Examples of such markers of differentiation include hemoglobin for mature red blood cells, prostate specific acid phosphatase for prostatic epithelial cells, lactalbumin for mammary cells, myoglobin for muscle cells etc. There are many steps in the pathway leading from DNA to protein; in principle, all of them can be regulated, affecting gene express-ions. These steps include: **transcriptional control** - when and how often a given gene is transcribed, **RNA processing control** - regulating how the RNA transcript is spliced, **RNA transport and localization control** – selecting the mRNAs to be exported from the nucleus to the cytoplasm and where in the cytoplasm they are to be localized, **translational control** – which mRNAs in the cytoplasm are translated, **mRNA degradation control** – selectively inactivating certain mRNA molecules in the cytoplasm, or **protein activity control**. For most genes, transcriptional control is the critical one.

These alterations in gene expressions can be [and often are] responses to external cues or stimuli; the signal(s) switching the regulatory regions of DNA near the site where transcription begins or by activating the gene regulatory proteins which turn genes on or off.

Figure 8-1 shows the effect of IP₆ on lactalbumin expression by human breast cancer cell line. Note that IP₆ treatment results in fewer cells (decreased proliferation) and increased differentiation.

Effect of IP₆ on breast cancer cells

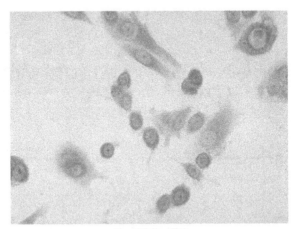

5 mM InsP6

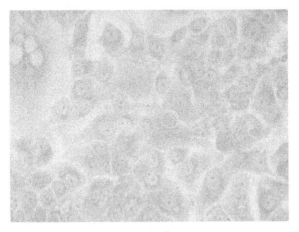

control

Figure 8-1: Upper panel shows increased lactalbumin as dark brown with associated decrease in cell number.

The bar-gram (Figure 8-2) shows that with increased doses of IP_6 there is increased lactalbumin expression (dose-response relationship).

Dose-Response Increase in Lactalbumin Production by IP_6

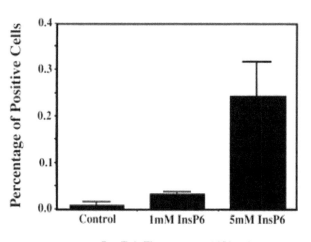

Figure 8-2: With higher dose of IP_6 more cells show normal behavioral pattern

IP_6 has been demonstrated to induce differentiation of malignant cells of divergent origins to the normal phenotype. It was first demonstrated in K-562 human erythroleukemia cells, which showed increased hemoglobin production following IP$_6$ treatment. Similar induction of tissue specific differentiation was reported for human colon carcinoma HT-29 cells, prostate cancer cells, breast cancer cells, and rhabdomyosarcoma cells. The molecular mechanisms involving these IP$_6$ - induced differentiation will be fascinating to study. It is however known that PI 3-K (phosphoinositide 3-kinase) plays an important role in granulocytic differentiation of HL-60 leukemia cells. Interestingly, the intracellular concentration of IP$_6$ and IP$_5$ is elevated by about two orders of magnitude during chemotactic stimulation of HL-60 cells. Clearly an elevated level of IP$_6$ plays a yet to be determined role in these differentiated functions.

Safeguarding our DNA

All living organisms grow and reproduce by means of cell division. Organisms that originally consisted of a single cell will see numerous cell divisions, each time generating so-called "daughter" cells. For instance, a fertilized human egg starts to divide and thus forms an embryo. As its cells divide over and over, it - in turn - will grow into a fetus. Even as adults, we must produce new cells continuously - millions and millions of them (approximately 10^{13} cells!). Some of our tissues and organs incessantly regenerate their cells by undergoing cell division. Some prime examples are our skin cells and the cells that line our digestive tract; our red blood cells (of which we need a steady new stream), and organs like the liver; it also demands ongoing "renovation work" (i.e., rebuilding).

Controlled Cell Growth

When unimpeded and functioning properly, cells divide under well regulated conditions: A cell divides and its resulting daughter cells start to develop. However, in situations where cell division becomes aberrant in some way – anomalous, excessive, or unfettered – a dangerous potential arises. Unrestrained cell division is seen as potential indication of cancer.

During the cell division process, most cells create an exact copy of their contents. At this point, the most vital prerequisite is an authentic and accurate replication of a cell's genetic material (i.e., of its DNA or deoxyribonucleic acid). The DNA is found inside the nucleus of the cell. The cell nucleus is separated from the other cellular contents by the surrounding membrane which serves to both isolate and shield the genetic material. Once the cell replication process has been completed, DNA is distributed to each of the daughter cells. This now makes the daughter cells a genetically identical copy of their parents' cells. In order to allow this genetic replication process the body must make fresh DNA.

DNA's building blocks consist of a chain of so-called "bases" - named as follows (the letters in parenthesis represent the symbols generally used to denote these bases): Adenine (A) - Guanine (G) - Cytosine (C) and Thymine (T). When these bases are linked together in a chain, a DNA strand is formed. A bulkier 2-ring base (a purine: adenine or guanine) is paired with a single ring pyrimidine base (cytosine or thymine). Here is an example where some bases are strung together in a particular sequence, thereby forming a specific strand of DNA: -A-G-C-T-G-A-C-T-, and so on, and so forth.

The different arrangements (i.e., sequences or configurations) of these base letters account for the genetic differences between various species of living organisms.

Within the DNA, we find two strands which are wound together and have their bases paired as follows:

- A is always paired with T;
- G is always paired with C.

This complementary base-pairing enables the base pairs (A=T or G=C) to be packed in the most favorable arrangement in the interior of the double helix. When the time has come for a cell to produce a copy of its DNA, the DNA strands, the double helix uncoil (unwind) and the new bases line up in such a way that they correspond to those on the original strand.

Specific bases within a group of cells can be radioactively tagged. This procedure makes it possible to determine the exact moment when the DNA synthesis occurs. The rate at which the DNA synthesis takes place can also be evaluated by measuring the quantity of the tagged bases that are being "processed".

A substance called thymidine (which combines the thiamine (T) base with a sugar molecule ribose) is used exclusively during the DNA synthesis process. We carried out experiments with radioactively marked thymidine (^{3}H-thymidine) which was incorporated into the DNA, after which we measured how much of the substance had been taken up.

Studies in my laboratory showed a suppression of DNA synthesis as measured by ^{3}H-thymidine incorporation and down-regulation of proliferation marker PCNA (proliferating cell nuclear antigen) by IP$_6$. A marked decrease in the expression of proliferation markers indicated that IP$_6$ disengaged cells from actively cycling. Using dual parameter flow cytometry and combined analysis of the expression of cell cycle-related proteins, we also demonstrated that IP$_6$ controls the progression of the cells through the cell cycle. IP$_6$ treatment significantly decreased the S-phase and arrested the human colon and breast cancer cells in the G$_0$/G$_1$ phase (El-Sherbiny *et al* 2001). Interestingly, the intracellular levels of IP$_6$ are high in G$_1$ and G$_2$/M phases of cell cycle, but drop by 50-75% during the S phase.

Studies of human leukemia cells at Prof. Lambertenghi-Deliliers' laboratory at the University of Milan demonstrate that IP$_6$ shows a dose-dependent cytotoxic effect on human leukemia cell lines. The IP$_6$-treated leukemia cells accumulate in G$_2$M phase of cell cycle (as opposed to G$_0$/G$_1$ phase in breast cancer cells); once again arrest of cells in the cycle, albeit in a different phase. Further investigation using cDNA micro array analysis showed an extensive down-modulation of genes involved in transcription and cell cycle regulation (c-myc, HPTPCAAX1, FUSE, cyclin H) and an upregulation of cell cycle inhibitors such as CKS2, p57 and Id-2. Genes such as STAT-6 and MAPKAP, involved in important signal transduction pathways were also down regulated.

DNA Damage

In order to continue our life form in this planet, all species must pass on the genetic information to the progeny, unchanged or unaltered. However, our DNA, the messenger (or carrier) of the information is under constant assault from physical and chemical agents both inside and outside our body. As if to counter that constant onslaught, life has evolved to not only detect, but also repair (within limits) the damages inflicted on the DNA. And every day, each of the approximately 10^{13} cells of our body ends up having tens of thousands of lesions in our DNA. These lesions can potentially 'send the wrong message' to the genome copies during DNA replication and then transcription. Of course, if these errors in the message are not corrected, or improperly corrected, they may result in gene mutation which may be catastrophically detrimental to the health of the cell, and even the organism. But fortunately, these damages are mostly not permanent and we have evolved to repair these damages, by and large. And the double helical structure of the DNA is ideally suited for repair as it carries two separate copies of all the genetic information; when one strand is damaged, the complementary strand retaining an intact copy of the same information is used to restore the correct nucleotide sequence and hence repair the damage. Single strand damages are less dangerous than double strand damage; the latter may be fatal to the cell. Ionizing radiation is a cause for double stranded DNA breaks. Aside from accidental (Chernobyl, Fukushima Daiichi), war-time (Hiroshima and Nagasaki) or terrorist-activated [feared] nuclear blast, one may find ionizing radiation in some homes as radioactive radon gas (from uranium decay) that contributes to lung cancer. We are also exposed to ionizing radiation from diagnostic and therapeutic agents such as technetium-99m (Tc^{99m}) iodine-131 (I^{131}) or cancer radiotherapy.

Fortunately, each cell contains many DNA repair systems, everyone with its own enzymes; most of these systems use the undamaged strand of the double helix (that contains a copy of the original information) as a template for repairing the damaged strand. Basically, for DNA with single strand damage, the damaged sequence is excised, the original sequence is restored by using the undamaged strand as template by the enzyme DNA polymerase and finally the break in the DNA is sealed by another enzyme, appropriately called DNA ligase. The various cancer-causing agents (carcinogens, such as those in tobacco products, fungal toxins as aflatoxins) as well as many of the cancer-treatment drugs (!) also damage DNA by forming adducts. The most pervasive of the environmental DNA damaging agents is ultraviolet (UV) light. Notwithstanding the increasing size of the hole, thanks to the ozone layer, the most dangerous part of the solar ultraviolet spectrum – UVC does not reach us. However, the residual UVA and UVB can induce approximately 100,000 DNA lesions/cell/day (Please see Review by Lord & Ashworth 2012). A common DNA lesion by UV radiation from sunlight is TT dimers produced by covalent linkage between two adjacent thymidine molecules in the DNA strand. If the lesion is not excised, the misinformation owing to abnormal base-pairing would lead to its substitution (mutation) in the daughter DNA chain during DNA replication. This mutation will then be propagated throughout subsequent generations of cells.

DNA Repair

As one would expect, to combat the various types of DNA damages there exists a rather elaborate maintenance/repair system for each category. For example, there are base-excision repair (BCR) removes the subtle modifications of DNA such as small base adduct. Bulkier single-strand lesions that distort the DNA helical structure (e.g. caused by UV light) are processed by nucleotide excision repair (NER). The double stranded breaks are handled through homologous recombination and non-homologous end joining (NHEJ); the latter – an imperfect process, simply brings two ends together wherein bases may be lost or added. Acting mainly during the S and G$_2$ phases of the cell cycle, homologous recombination on the other hand tends to restore the original DNA sequence.

Let's look at how IP$_6$ and inositol can help. As mentioned before, double strand breaks are potentially dangerous as you can imagine - that if left unrepaired, they may cause the chromosomes to break into small fragments and eventually to cell death. This type of damage is caused by ionizing radiation, oxidizing agents etc. IP_6 has been demonstrated to stimulate non-homologous end-joining; it has been proposed to be brought about by the binding of IP_6 to the DNA-dependent protein kinase DNA-PK_{cs}. Detailed study show that it is not DNA-PK_{cs} (a large protein of ~3500 amino acids, M_w ~465 kDa), but the DNA end binding protein Ku (consists of Ku70 - 70 kDa, and Ku86 - 83 kDa) that binds to IP_6. IP_6 has a potent effect on mobility and dynamics of Ku through a region of Ku70. Recent studies show that Ku is precisely regulated by binding to IP_6 and activation of DNA-PK plays a key role in non-homologous end-joining repair. Be that as it may, these studies, despite their differences in their specific findings clearly show a very important role of IP_6 in DNA repair mechanism.

Once the assault on the cell has gone past the scope of DNA repair, the otherwise heretofore normal cell is likely to transform to a malignant (cancer) cell. Insofar as the transformation of cells from normal to malignancy is concerned, there are various models and pathways, one of these pathways is the activation of transcription factors activating protein-1 (AP-1) and nuclear factor NFκB *via* phosphatidylinositol 3-kinase (PI-3 kinase). Using tumor promoter-induced cell transformation of human skin JB6 cells, Huang *et al* (1997) have demonstrated that IP$_6$ blocks epidermal growth factor-induced PI-3 kinase and AP-1 activity. That IP$_6$ also acts as an anti-mutagenic agent has been recently demonstrated by Ra Yoon *et al* (2008).

DNA damage is also caused by reactive oxygen compounds arising as byproducts of oxidative respiration or from environmental toxic agents. We will discuss that in the next chapter.

Telomerase

The ends of the DNA strands are identified as 3' or 5'. At the 3' end of all vertebrate DNA exists nucleotide repeat sequences TTAGGG, the region is called telomere. This segment of DNA is non-coding and essentially caps (protects the DNA from losing important coding sequences) the coding segments. With each cell division, there is shortening of the telomere. Telomerase (the subject of 2009 Nobel Prize in Physiology & Medicine) elongates the shortened telomere without which important DNA message will be lost. Since the activation of telomerase is crucial for cells to gain immortality and proliferation ability, Jagadeesh &

Banerjee (2006) examined the role of IP_6 in the regulation of telomerase activity in murine and human prostate cancer cells. They demonstrate that IP_6 represses telomerase activity in prostate cancer cells in a dose-dependent manner. In addition, they show that IP_6 prevents the translocation of TERT (telomerase reverse transcriptase) to the nucleus and inhibits phosphorylation of Akt and PKCα. Thus, IP_6 represses telomerase activity in prostate cancer cells by post-translational modification of TERT *via* deactivation of Akt and PKCα. Using human glioblastoma T98G cell line, Karmakar *et al* (2007) also demonstrated the repression of telomerase activity by IP_6. An important point to keep in mind is that the telomerase activity may have conflicting roles – truncated telomeres can be seen as harbinger of both good and bad; research will tell us more.

Epigenetic changes

The early steps in carcinogenesis involving gene expression without affecting DNA sequence modification are no less important. DNA methyl transferases, methyl CpG binding proteins, methyl CpG DNA binding domain protein, and histone deacetylases are the major molecules involved in epigenetics. In the December 2010 issue of the Journal *Nutrition & Cancer* Drs. Pandey and Gupta report that in their mouse-lung tumorigenesis model, while the carcinogen ENU up-regulated the epigenetic events such as the expressions of DNMT1, MeCP2, MBD1, and HDAC1, these alterations were reduced by IP_6 administration.

Angiogenesis

Because angiogenesis depends on the interaction between endothelial and tumor cells, we investigated the effect of IP_6 on both the cell types (Vucenik *et al* 2004). IP_6 inhibited the proliferation and induced the differentiation of endothelial cells *in vitro*; the growth of bovine aortic endothelial cells (BAECs) evaluated by MTT proliferation assay was inhibited in a dose-dependent manner (IC_{50} = 0.74 mM). The combination of IP_6 and vasostatin, a calreticulin fragment with anti-angiogenic activity was synergistically superior in growth inhibition than either compound. IP_6 inhibited human umbilical vein endothelial cell (HUVEC) tube formation (*in vitro* capillary differentiation) on a reconstituted extracellular matrix, Matrigel, and disrupted preformed tubes. IP_6 significantly reduced basic fibroblast growth factor (bFGF)-induced vessel formation ($p < 0.01$) *in vivo* in Matrigel plug assay.

For our experiments on the other component cells – the cancer cells, we chose HepG2 cells. Exposure of HepG2, a human hepatoma cell line, to IP₆ for 8 h, resulted in a dose-dependent decrease in the mRNA levels of vascular endothelial growth factor (VEGF), as assessed by RT-PCR. IP₆ treatment of HepG2 cells for 24 h also significantly reduced the VEGF protein levels in conditioned medium, in a concentration-dependent manner ($p = 0.012$). These data show that IP₆'s anti-angiogenesis action is directed towards both the endothelial cells and the cancer cells.

Prof. Agarwal's laboratory has been working with prostate cancer. DU145 prostate cancer cells were injected into nude mice, and animals were fed normal drinking water or 1 or 2% IP₆ in drinking water for 12 weeks and the tumors were analyzed for proliferating cell nuclear antigen, terminal deoxynucleotidyl transferase-mediated nick end labeling, and CD31. Tumor-secreted insulin-like growth factor binding protein (IGF-BP)-3 and VEGF were quantified in plasma. IP₆ feeding of the animals resulted in suppression of hormone-refractory human prostate tumor growth without any adverse effect on body weight gain, diet, and water consumption during entire study. There was a dose-response inhibition of tumor growth: at the end of study, tumor growth inhibition by 1 and 2% IP_6 feeding was 47 and 66% ($p = 0.049$-0.012) in terms of tumor volume/mouse and 40 and 66% ($p = 0.08$-0.003) in terms of tumor weight/mouse, respectively. Tumor xenografts from IP_6-fed mice showed significantly ($p < 0.001$) decreased proliferating cell nuclear antigen-positive cells but increased apoptotic cells. Tumor-secreted IGFBP-3 levels were also increased up to 1.7-fold in IP_6-fed groups. Furthermore, IP_6 strongly decreased tumor micro-vessel density and inhibited tumor-secreted VEGF levels.

CHAPTER 9

ANTIOXIDANT
MECHANISM OF
ACTION II

Antioxidant Protection

As we have seen, IP$_6$ plays many different roles;
however, many of its favorable health impacts can
be traced back to its function as an antioxidant. Before I discuss IP$_6$'s antioxidative properties in
more detail, we first need to review what exactly
an antioxidant is and what does such a substance

"work against"; in other words, why is it called an **anti**-oxidant)?

Oxygen is obviously indispensable for human life (and for the existence of most other organisms). However, as paramount as its role is for our well-being, once inside the human body, there needs to be a strict regulation of quantities and specific activities. The reason for this is that an excess of oxygen can cause substantial damage to our cells and their intracellular components (the complex and delicate "machinery" at work inside our cells). The molecule's chemical symbol "O_2" indicates that two oxygen atoms are bonded together.

When molecules that contain oxygen interact with each other in certain chemical reactions so-called "free radicals" may be produced. As you might recall from your science classes, electrons are electrically charged particles that circle around the center (nucleus) of an atom. Atoms can take on different energy configurations – when we see electrons appear in pairs, the atom is considered to be in its "most favored state" in terms of energy. In situations where each molecule of oxygen has an equal number of shared electrons, it is in a "content" state. "Discontent" may however arise if one of the electrons is pulled away from the molecule, thus leaving the other unpaired. (Molecules are the smallest units of chemical compounds consisting of two or more atoms). What happens in the "discontent stage" is that the "free" or unpaired electron will endeavor to secure another oxygen molecule's electron so that it may form a new electron pairing. When an atom or a molecule has an unpaired electron, and is thus in a state where it seeks to acquire electrons from other atoms or molecules, it is called a free radical.

A particular type of free radical is an energy-laden, highly reactive form of oxygen called "singlet oxygen" - written as "$O_2.-$".

The dot in this formula denotes the presence of an unpaired electron. This gives the singlet oxygen a net negative charge – a fact indicated by the use of the negative ("-") sign in the above formula. Two other names for singlet oxygen are "activated oxygen" or "reactive oxygen species".

Singlet oxygen is just one of many known free radicals. Two other examples of free radicals are:

1. Hydrogen peroxide (H_2O_2) – it has two unpaired electrons;

2. The hydroxyl radical (•OH) – it has three unpaired electrons.

Both of the above reactive species are members of a group called the superoxides. Superoxides may cause damage to one's DNA, to proteins, as well as to other cell components. The fundamental chemical reaction underlying such damage is called an oxidation reaction. The free radicals produced in such a process are called oxidants. Aside from the environmental toxic agents (both physical and chemical) that produce oxygen free radicals, reactive oxygen and nitrogen compounds are also formed by the macrophages and polymorphonuclear leukocytes at the site of inflammation and infection. In the DNA, these chemicals can cause adduct formation that can impair the ability of DNA for correct base pairing. And that's not all. The DNA replication and transcription may be blocked, nucleotides may be lost or there may even be DNA single strand breaks.

Antioxidants received their name from the fact that they can fight oxidants; in other words, they are "anti" the oxidants.

How do antioxidants stop oxidants? They do so by supplying oxidants with the missing electrons they seek (as outlined above). In this way, antioxidants are able to prevent oxidative chain reactions which can induce cellular damage.

A number of antioxidants are widely known; you may have heard of the following:

- Vitamin C (ascorbate);
- The vitamin E family (tocopherols);
- Substances like β-carotene and lycopene

And both inositol and IP$_6$ are also antioxidants, IP$_6$ being one of the most powerful.

Let's look further at free radicals. Interestingly, free radicals do not always pose a threat to our health; they also have properties that can be very beneficial. For instance, free radicals can be produced by neutrophils – a particular type of white blood cells that serves the immune system by engulfing invaders (such as bacteria) which have managed to penetrate the body's first line of defense. Neutrophils use superoxides (and other free radicals) to kill invaders they have trapped. Within the neutrophils, we find tiny "sacs" which store these oxidants until they are needed. The safe storage of free radicals in this fashion ensures that they cannot damage cell structures; as well, the free radicals are not inadvertently rendered inactive by antioxidants – they are stored until ready to be dropped like bombs on the enemy. The body must handle free radicals with great care because they are like a double-edged sword. While they serve to fulfill vital protective functions within our immune system, an excessive or otherwise abnormal buildup of free radicals could be very damaging to the host – which in this case is us.

But free radicals are not just generated within our bodies; numerous external sources produce them as well. Here are just a few potent examples:

- Cigarette smoke;
- The sun's UV radiation;
- Indiscriminate use of oxygen therapy;
- Radiation from cancer therapy;
- Drugs;
- Our everyday diet. It, too, can generate free radicals during the food metabolism.

Free radicals can damage our DNA. This so-called oxidative damage to our genetic material can then generate mutations, which in turn may promote a wide array of diseases, from cataracts to cancers. At least in part, free radicals can also contribute directly to the aging process.

If a cell has sustained DNA damage, and if that damage is not repaired, the cell may be prevented from replicating or copying its own DNA. In cases where a cell does not need to divide, the consequences may be benign. However, we have many cells that must divide – if they are prevented from doing so (i.e., if their DNA cannot be replicated), the consequences can be far direr: Cell death can be the result. Under normal circumstances, enzymes naturally found in our bodies are able to cut out (excise) those parts of a DNA strand that have sustained oxidative damage. This repair mechanism can however become undermined when the DNA mutations caused by oxidative damage accumulate over time as they tend to. Serious health problems - cancers and other diseases commonly associated with the aging process can be the result.

In 1993, Dr. Bruce Ames and his colleagues reported on research performed on the topic of free radicals and aging. They discovered – as other scientists have - that specific diseases and the aging process in general tend to accelerate when cells and their DNA are not adequately protected by antioxidants.

How does IP₆ function as antioxidant?

To understand this, we must discuss the mito-chondria – the plentiful tiny cellular structures that have been called the cells' "energy factories". Within the mitochondria, a complex series of che-mical reactions takes place, further processing compounds originating from our diet. The end res-ult of these reactions is the extraction of energy that ultimately sustains us. This miraculous pro-cess that turns metabolic fuel into actual energy is called "respiration". Please note that the word in this context does not have the same meaning as the term applied to the process of breathing.

Respiration at the cellular level takes place within the mitochondria; it involves the transference of electrons from molecule to molecule. During this reaction, it is critically important that the mineral iron be present. Cells procure the iron they need from the blood plasma. During the respiration pro-cess, free radicals are generated as a byproduct. Whereas some of these free radicals are in fact necessary for the respiration itself, an excessive production of reactive species represents a dangerous potential. In a process called the Fenton reaction, hydrogen peroxide (H_2O_2) is formed. The H_2O_2 then reacts with the iron, sparking the production of highly reactive and damaging hydroxyl radicals ($\bullet OH$).

At the site of the Fenton reaction, IP_6 binds to excess iron, thus inhibiting the formation of hydroxyl radicals. IP_6's activity in this regard is highly beneficial, because it prevents an ensuing (and harmful) reaction from taking place, the so-called lipid peroxidation. Lipid peroxidation is a type of damage sustained by the fats (lipids) that are natural constituents of cell membranes where membrane lipids come under attack by free radicals. Our cell membranes have embedded molecules called phospholipids which are produced from fatty acids and phosphates. Phosphatidyl inositol biphosphate (PIP2) is an example of such a phospholipid.

IP_6's antioxidant properties also protect DNA from the ravages of free radicals. As discussed earlier, IP_6 has the ability to chelate (i.e. bind) iron, consequently suppressing the production of oxygen free radicals.

Though the antioxidant property of IP_6 has been known since the mid 1979's, I wanted to study it myself just for my edification. To that effect, Dr. Mary J. Hinzman and Dr. Peter L. Gutierrez - two of my colleagues at the University of Maryland School of Medicine – conducted an experiment where they applied a technique called electron spin resonance spectroscopy. They were able to demonstrate that IP_6 has the capacity to reduce the formation of free radicals. In fact, once IP_6 was added, free radical production dropped by more than a factor of 2.5. By virtue of its antioxidative powers, IP_6 reduced the active oxygen species-mediated cancer formation and cell injury.

In a later chapter, I shall discuss a common example where lung destruction is caused by asbestos. It will prove conclusively how IP_6 can stop the damaging effects of free radicals.

IP_6's oxidative capacities also come into play in the plant kingdom. Here, IP_6 serves to preserve and protect seeds, allowing them to remain viable and keep their ability to grow for extended periods of time.

Inositol as an Antioxidant

Inositol has also been demonstrated to have anti-oxidative properties. Drs. S. Muraoka and T. Miura from Hokkaido College of Pharmacy in Otaru, Japan, reported in the February 13, 2004 issue of the journal *Life Sciences* (volume 74: pages 1691-1700, 2004) that not only IP₆, but inositol also inhibits xanthine oxidase induced superoxide dependent DNA damage. Though not entirely clear as to how, their data suggest that inositol may also act as hydroxyl radical scavenger!

In an inter-American collaborative study from several institutions in Ceará, Brazil and New York and Philadelphia in U.S.A, Dr. Nascimento and collaborators showed that inositol exerts its anti-oxidant function by inhibiting xanthine oxidase and scavenging superoxide both *in vitro* and *in vivo*, and preventing formation of ADP-iron-oxygen complexes that initiate lipid peroxidation ("Inositols prevents and reverse endothelial dysfunction in diabetic rat and rabbit vasculature metabolically and by scavenging superoxide": *Proceedings of the National Academy of Sciences USA*, volume 103: pages 218-223, January 2006). This is the basis for prevention and even reversal of endothelial cell dysfunction in diabetes. How is that significant? A markedly increased risk of cardiovascular diseases is seen in diabetes. These include myocardial infarction, stroke, peripheral vascular disease – resulting in amputation of limbs, etc. All of these are causally related to the abnormal functionality of endothelial cells (cells lining the inner wall of our blood vessels).

Lee *et al* (2005) have dissected out the mechanism of IP_6±inositol-induced suppression of liver cancer by using a rat hepatocarcinogenesis model initiated by diethylnitrosamine (DEN) and promoted by partial hepatectomy (PH). Supplementation with either inositol or IP_6, or their combination resulted in a significant decrease in both the area and the number of placental glutathione S transferase positive (GST-P+) foci, a marker of preneoplastic changes in DEN-initiated hepatocarcinogenesis. The administration of IP_6±inositol in drinking water caused marked enhancement in the glutathione S-transferase (GST) activity. In addition, the production of thiobarbituric acid reactive substances and the catalase activity were significantly reduced in rats supplemented with IP_6 ± inositol. Thus, the chemopreventive effects of IP_6± inositol on rat hepatocarcinogenesis, at least in this model initiated by DEN and promoted by PH, are associated with induction of GST activity and sup-perssion of lipid peroxidation.

In summary, the protective benefits exerted by IP_6 and inositol as antioxidants extend to diabetes, cancer, cardiovascular diseases, cataracts, just to name a few. And, given the synergistic function of IP_6 and inositol in providing the best anticancer action the cocktail: IP_6+Inositol is the most effective, safe and promises a wide spectrum of health benefits.

IP₆ Citrate - The Super Antioxidant

A new IP_6 molecule has been created: Addition of citrate to IP_6 molecule gives rise to a new molecule called inositol hexaphosphate citrate (IP_{6c}). While the parent IP_6 molecule has 12 valences, the new one (IP_{6c}) has 24, making it a better chelator and hence an even better antioxidant, perhaps the strongest available to date.

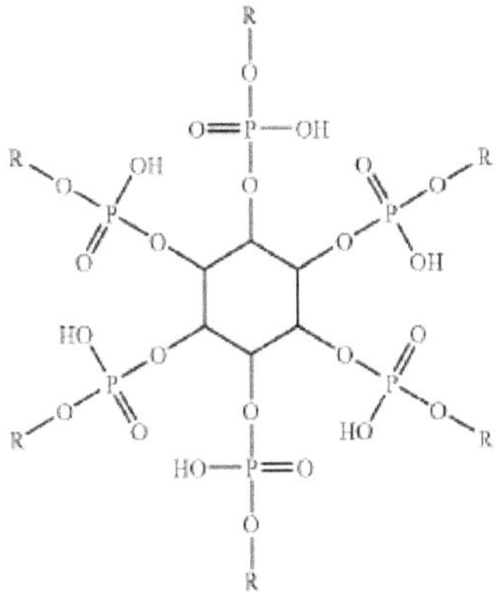

Figure 9-1: IP₆ Citrate; each R can be either H or Citrate, thus there could be IP₆Cit₁₋₆

Approximately 75% of the phosphates in the feed for cattle, pigs and poultry are from IP₆ in corn seed. Non-ruminants such as poultry and pigs do not have efficient enzyme system to utilize that phosphate resulting in environmental problems such as water pollution and eutrophication with decreased bone phosphates in the animals themselves; addition of citric acid to the feed improves that "phytate-phosphorous" utilization (Abelson PH. 1999; Rafacz-Livingston *et al* 1999). Thus, the new molecule, phytic citrate or IP₆Cit could be an important improvement that is likely to be not only healthy for the cattle, pigs

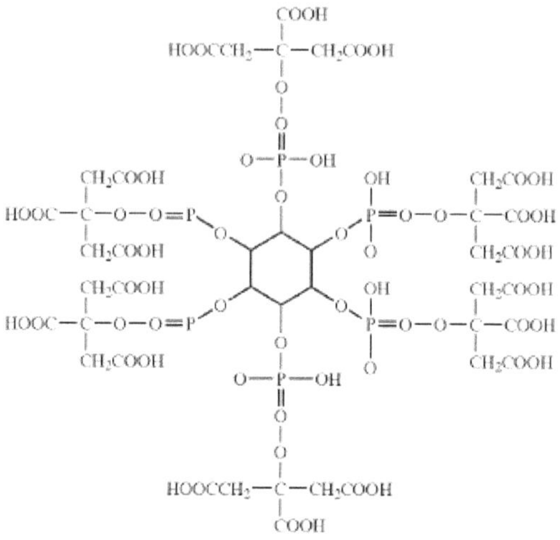

Figure 9-2: Hexacitrated IP₆

and poultry, but also provide better environment. And, our preliminary data [unpublished results] indicate that, indeed, IP_6Cit may be more potent in cancer inhibition than IP_6.

It seems that IP_6 is the perennial scapegoat of them, all. While some are quick to blame IP_6 phosphate for eutrophication (increased nutrient initially causing increased productivity such as crops, followed by environmental damages as poor water quality, overgrowth of algae etc.), the overwhelming contribution by phosphates from fertilizers is often neglected. As a matter of fact, the phosphate from IP$_6$ in the manure can be the answer to some our environmental problems. Please see the article "The Disappearing Nutrient" by Natasha Gilbert in *Nature* **461**:716-718, 8 October 2009.

CHAPTER 10

IMMUNE SUPPORT
&
INFLAMMATION

Our Defense Systems

Plants and animals have to continually defend themselves from invaders – viruses, bacteria, fungi, parasites etc. The defense mechanisms are classified as either natural or acquired. The engulfing (phagocytosis) of bacteria by polymorphonuclear leukocytes (also known as neutrophils) and mono-cytes in our blood or by tissue macrophages is an example of *natural defense or immunity*. The en-gulfed bacteria are then digested by the enzyme that literally comes in packets – lysosomal granu-les. Actual killing of the invading bacteria or fungi is done by activated oxygen species – hydroxyl radicals ($\bullet OH$) that are produced through a series of activities that converts molecular oxygen (O_2) to the superoxide anion O_2^-; these intracellular activities are known together as "respiratory burst." There is non-oxidative killing as well *via* a variety of enzyme systems. Thus, the process of inflamm-ation and associated reaction by the army of cells standing by, is our immediate natural defense. This natural immunity neither requires prior exposure to the offender or invader, nor is it enhanced by such experience. It is also non-specific, that is, it does not (or cannot) discriminate among the vari-ous offenders who are essentially foreign.

Acquired Immunity, by contrast is specific, requi-res a sensitizing exposure to the invader or offen-der and subsequent encounters magnifies the resp-onse. The cellular components of acquired immu-nity are the T lymphocytes, B lymphocytes, natu-ral killer (NK) cells and mononuclear phagocytes.

Natural Killer (NK) Cells

The thymus-derived T cells constitute 60-70% of
the peripheral blood lymphocytes, B cells 10-20%
and the natural killer (NK) cells 10-15%. NK cells
are somewhat larger than small lymphocytes and
have also been called large granular lymphocytes.
The NK cells have an inherent ability to destroy
virally infected cells and a variety of tumor cells,
and some normal cells. This ability to lyse cells is
innate and is not dependent on prior sensitization
or experience; this ability is *natural* and forms the
first line of defense against cancer or viral infections; however, they may be stimulated by various
cytokines such as interferon (INFα/β and inter-
leukin 2 (IL2). NK cells contain special weaponry
- perforin and proteases known as granzymes. As
the name suggests, perforin punches holes (perfo-
rates) the target cells through which the granzymes
and associated molecules enter and cause cell death.

I shall now address IP₆'s response to each of the
preceding items in the order they were discussed
above.

IP₆ Boosts Our Natural Defense

The polymorphonuclear leukocytes (or more simply: Neutrophils) are capable of destroying bacteria; however, as stated earlier, they first require
stimulation in the form of a so-called respiratory
burst - a series of chemical events that allows the
neutrophils to generate free radicals capable of
killing the bacteria. In connection with IP₆, an
interesting discovery was made by Dr. Paul Eggleton, who is now at the Universities of Exeter and
Plymouth in England. In 1991, he and his colleagues found that human polymorphonuclear leukocytes – when preincubated with IP₆ had a greatly
augmented capacity to produce reactive oxygen
species (when the leukocytes were stimulated either by chemicals or by the presence of bacteria). Dr.
Eggleton's conclusion was that the resulting improvement in host defense was yet another beneficial function attributable to IP₆. Paradoxically,
while IP₆ acts as a rather potent antioxidant in most
other instances, herein, it enhances the ability of
polymorphonuclear leukocytes to produce more
superoxide so that they can kill the bacteria, and
more efficiently!

Macrophage

Realizing the paucity of data on IP_6's ability to enhance the natural disease resistance of the body, Dr. M. Johnson and colleagues at the University of Mississippi, Jackson embarked on a study to investigate the effects of IP_6 on the proliferation and viability of RAW 264.7 transformed macrophages and to investigate the role of IP_6 as a free radical scavenger. They report that the rate of cell proliferation of the macrophages was totally dependent on the dose of IP_6. Their results suggest that IP_6 have an excitatory effect on the inflammatory cell secretions which is dose-dependent.

We are fortunate to have many other innate defenses in our body; one of these is the intestinal lining epithelial cells. Aside from forming a mechanical barrier directly separating our interior from the luminal contents, they also are actively involved in the local immune response team. The cytokine IL-8 (interleukin-8) attracts the neutrophils (chemotaxis), causes them to release the deadly oxygen free radicals and enzymes to combat the intruder. IL-6 too is involved in inflammatory response in addition to being part of the normal immune response. A recent study by Prof. Ludmiła Węglarz *et al* from the Medical University of Silesia, Pol-

and suggest that IP_6 may exert immunoregulatory effects on colonic epithelium to maintain it in a rather healthy non-inflammatory state or to counteract infection, by modulating the release of the cytokine IL-8 and IL-6, the interleukins.

IP₆ Tackles Inflammation and Fibrosis

Gastric Ulcer

Dr. Sudheer Kumar and colleagues from the College of Pharmaceutical Sciences, Manipal India, investigated the effect of IP_6 in experimental models of inflammation and gastric ulcer. In the carrageenan-induced rat paw edema model they observed an anti-inflammatory activity of IP_6, maximum at an oral dose of 150 mg/kg. IP_6 showed an ability to prevent denaturation of proteins but it showed less anti-inflammatory activity than ibuprofen (albeit without sharing the side-effects of ibuprofen!). The researchers believe that the ability of IP_6 to bring down thermal denaturation of proteins might be a contributing factor in the mechanism of action against inflammation. *IP₆ at all the doses tested, showed significant protection from ulcers induced by ibuprofen, ethanol and cold stress*. There was a significant increase in gastric tissue malondialdehyde levels in ethanol treated rats but these levels decreased following IP$_6$ pretreatment. Moreover, pretreatment with IP$_6$ significantly inhibited various effects of ethanol on gastric mucosa, such as, reduction in the concentration of non-protein sulfhydryl groups, necrosis, erosions, congestion and hemorrhage. Thus, the gastro-protective effect of IP$_6$ could be mediated by its antioxidant activity and cytoprotection of gastric mucosa.

Asbestosis

It is a well-established fact that exposure to asbestos can lead to fibrosis – the formation of fibrous (scar) tissue in response to an irritant – and to lung cancer. It is believed that oxidative damage (for instance caused by superoxide free radicals) is an early, key contributor in a sequence of chemical events that leads to asbestos-induced damage of the lungs. Several mechanisms appear to play a role, among them:

- Inflammation triggered by asbestos leads to a production of superoxides;

- The earlier discussed Fenton reaction may also play a role in that the iron present in the asbestos can catalyze the formation of superoxides.

What is IP_6's role in this? Given its capacity to get rid of iron, as well as its ability to incapacitate free radicals, IP_6 can diminish the tissue damage sustained from such inflammatory processes.

In experiments where animals were exposed to asbestos have revealed that IP_6 can:

- Suppress the formation of superoxide free radicals;

- Reduce DNA damage;

- Lower the degree of inflammation and the extent of subsequent lung fibrosis.

In a 1995 paper on experiments carried out at the Northwestern University Medical School and Veterans Affair Lakeside Medical Center in Chicago, Dr. David Kamp and his colleagues exposed rats to asbestos. Two groups of experimental animals were studied – a group of rats receiving IP_6, and a control group not given any. As the researchers had anticipated, asbestos exposure induced a severe inflammatory and fibrotic reaction in the animals' lungs; however, the treatment with IP_6 was able to mitigate the damage in a statistically significant way. The degree of inflammation and fibrosis induced by the asbestos exposure was reduced anywhere from a factor of 6 to 36! Based on these study findings, it is conceivable that we might develop strategies using IP_6 to restrict the amount of asbestos-induced damage in humans known to be at high risk.

Dr. Kemp and associates having previously demonstrated that IP_6 reduces amosite asbestos-induced •OH generation, DNA strand-break formation, and injury to cultured pulmonary epithelial cells (1995) they then set out to determine whether IP_6 diminishes pulmonary inflammation and fibrosis in rats after a single intra-tracheal instillation of amosite asbestos. Sprague-Dawley rats were given either saline, amosite asbestos (5 mg; 1 ml saline), or amosite treated with IP_6 (500 μM) for 24 hr. At various times after asbestos exposure, the rats were euthanized and the lungs were lavaged and examined histologically. A fibrosis score was determined by special staining. Compared to controls, asbestos elicited a significant pulmonary inflammatory response, as evidenced by an approximately 2-fold increase in bronchoalveolar lavage (BAL) cell counts and the percentage of BAL neutrophils and giant cells at 2 wk (0.1 v 6.5% and 1.3 v 6.1%, respectively); the results being statistically significant at $p < 0.05$. Compared to asbestos alone, IP₆-treated asbestos elicited significantly less BAL PMNs (6.5 v 1.0%; p < 0.05) and giant cells (6.1 v 0.2%; $p < 0.05$) and caused significantly less fibrosis (5 v 0.8; $p < 0.05$) 2 wk after exposure. This study most convincingly demonstrates that asbestos cause pulmonary inflammation and fibrosis in rats and IP₆ clearly reduces these effects.

Giving NK Cells a Boost

Another important function of IP₆ is its involvement in the regulation of cellular resistance (immunity). I already mentioned natural killer (NK) cells, which play a pivotal role in the body's immune system. In 1980, Dr. Abdul Baten - a young doctor from Bangladesh who completed his M.D. and Ph.D. in Moscow, Russia – joined my laboratory and displayed great enthusiasm for my research. Because NK cells were his field of expertise, we decided to investigate together whether the anticancer (antineoplastic) properties of IP₆ could be attributed to the action of NK cells; it is a well-known fact that NK cells are important in fighting tumors. In our experiment, we used a mouse lymphoma (i.e., a cancer of the lymph gland) cell line named YAC-1 as the target cells on which to test the cytotoxicity (i.e., the cell-killing ability) of mouse spleen natural killer cells. We found that those mice who had developed carcinogen-induced tumors but had been treated *in vivo* with IP$_6$, displayed significantly enhanced NK cell activity (compared to the untreated control animals). The NK activity correlated positively with the extent of the tumor suppression; in other words, an increase in NK activity was associated with a lower incidence of cancer (Baten et al., 1989). When spleenocytes from healthy mice were treated *in vitro* with IP$_6$, the activity of the natural killer cells was also markedly increased (please see Figure 10-1 and 10-2).

The question now arises, what can IP$_6$ do to raise defenses in a ***human*** host? Dr. Ivana Vucenik – a

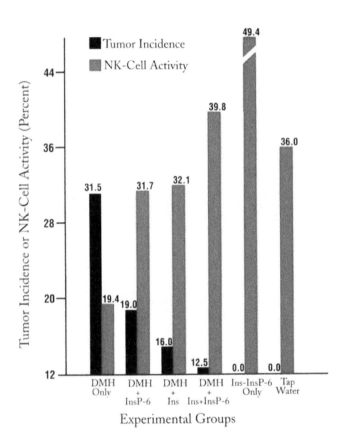

Figure 10-1: DMH: 1, 2-dimethyl hydrazine, InsP₆: IP₆, Ins: inositol. Note that the Ins-InsP₆ ONLY group did not have induced tumor (0.0) and their NK activity was the highest (49.4%), more than tap water control.

hematologist from Croatia also took an interest in our work and began to study this issue.

Wishing to investigate the NK activity specifically in humans, she carried out several experiments with

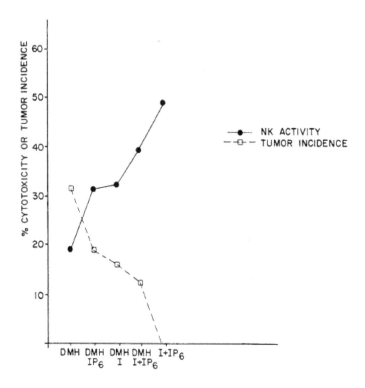

Figure 10-2: Note that as the NK activity is boosted by IP₆ ±Inositol the incidence of tumor goes down.

human NK cells – including some samples from her own blood. Dr Vucenik found that IP₆+inositol raises the natural killer cells' capacity to destroy human tumor cells. Thus, we had shown that IP_6+inositol markedly boosts NK cell activity both in mice and in humans. Our preliminary experiments to prove the same in rats were inconclusive. However, nearly two decades later, Drs. Z. Zhang, Y. Song and X-L. Wang from Qingdao University Medical School (home of the famous Chinese beer Ching-Tao!), reported a similar correlation in rats, concomitant to a decreased number and size of tumors as well as reduced metastasis, IP_6 also boosted the NK cell activity in yet another species – the rats

HIV

Every now and then, an event occurs that converts even the greatest skeptics into believers! Such circumstance occurred in 1989. Dr. Toru Otake and his colleagues from the Osaka Prefectural Institute of Public Health and Tottori University in Japan were able to show that, to a moderate degree, IP_6 could restrain the destructive (cytopathic) forces exerted by the human immunodeficiency virus (HIV), which causes AIDS. The experiment was carried out using MT-4 cells – an HIV susceptible cell line. Further results from Dr. Otake's work suggest that IP_6 also inhibited the HIV-specific antigen expression.

My colleague Dr. H.C. Tran *et al* (2003) at the University of Maryland Biotechnology Institute and the School of Medicine in Baltimore presented data at the 94th Annual Meeting of the American Association for Cancer Research in Washington D.C. that IP_6 blocks the tumorigenesis and angio-genic potential in both AIDS/Iatrogenic Kaposi's sarcoma and adult T-cell lymphoma cells *in vitro*.

This work has not been expanded, but there are at least two intriguing papers on the role of IP_6 in HIV viral particle assembly (Campbell *et al* 2001, Datta *et al* 2007).

In conclusion: We know that IP_6 enhances NK cell activity and that it stimulates the polymorphonu-clear cell priming function. Additionally, we can now surmise that IP_6 may find beneficial appli-cations in the management of HIV infections and associated immunodeficiency-linked complicati-ons.

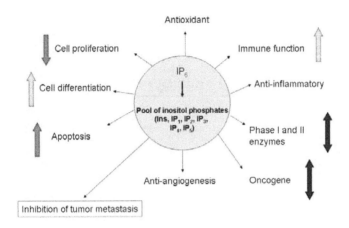

Figure 10-3: Summary of the mechanisms of action of IP₆

The above schematic diagram summarizes the various possible broad mechanisms of action of IP₆ that we have learnt so far. With more research, we will be able to discern perhaps additional modes of action with potential discovery of added benefits.

CHAPTER 11

RADIATION

PROTECTION

Radiation is energy distributed across the electro-magnetic spectrum, interacting with matter in a way that may be described by reference to waves (having long wavelength and low frequency) and/or to particles (having short wavelength and high frequency). Approximately 80% of all radiation encountered normally by mammals is from naturally-occurring sources. Radiation, particularly ionizing radiation, has an adverse effect on cells and tissues, primarily through cytotoxic effects. In humans, exposure to ionizing radiation occurs primarily through therapeutic techniques (such as anticancer radiotherapy), through occupational and/or environmental exposure to human-derived radiation sources, or through occupational exposure to naturally-occurring radiation sources as in the case of aircraft flight personnel.

Ionizing radiation is characterized as having short wavelength and high frequency; typical ionizing radiation forms include ultraviolet light, X-rays, gamma rays and cosmic radiation. Forms of ionizing radiation also include radioactive emissions of particles such as alpha particles or neutrons. In accord with its particulate nature, ionizing radiation causes vibration and rotation of atoms in biological molecules resulting in the ejection of electrons and the creation of free radicals. As discussed before, free radicals have a single unpaired electron in an outer orbit. This unstable configuration favors the release of energy through interactions with neighboring molecules, both inorganic and organic. In biological molecules, this rele-

ase results in physical alteration of molecules through the creation of aberrant chemical bonds.

Table 11-1 characterizes radiation forms according to their frequency and selected biological effects.

Table 11-1: Ionizing and Non-Ionizing Electromagnetic Radiation

Radiation	Frequency (Hz)	Biological Effects
Electrical power	1-50	?Increased incidence of cancer
Radio waves and radar	106-1,011	Thermal effects, cataract
Microwaves	109-1,010	Lens opacities
Infrared	1,011-1,014	Cataracts
Visible lights (lasers)	1,015	Retinal burns
Ultraviolet light	1,015-1,018	Skin burns, Skin cancer
X-rays and gamma rays	1,018-1,020	Acute and delayed injury, cancer
Cosmic radiation	1,027	?cataract, brain damage, cancer

Properties of radiation forms closer to the low-fre-
quency end of the spectrum are better described as

wavelike. Radiation forms closer to the high-frequency end of the spectrum have the most energy and tend to interact with matter as particles. The hazardous effects of radiation exposure are typically associated with the particulate characteristics of the radiation type.

Radiation Damage

Free radical species may also be created through chemical, enzymatic, and catalytic means by way of an intermediate reactive substance, but ionizing radiation can create free radicals directly, for example by directly hydrolyzing water into hydroxyl (•OH) and hydrogen (•H) free radicals. For example, when tissues are exposed to gamma radiation, much of the energy deposited in the cells is absorbed by water and results in scission of the oxygen-hydrogen covalent bonds in water, leaving a single electron on hydrogen and another on oxygen, thus creating the two radicals. The hydroxyl radical (•OH) is the most reactive radical known in chemistry.

As discussed earlier, free radical species react with the purine or pyrimidine bases of nucleic acids, proteins, lipids, and other biological micromolecules to produce damage to cells and tissues, and they can set off intra- and extracellular chain reactions, particularly in the critically ill patient. For example, reactive free-radical oxygen species initiate the activation of transcription factors through signal transduction from the cell surfaces, resulting in inflammation and tumor promotion.

DNA is the crucial target for the cytotoxic effects of ionizing radiation. Ionizing radiation is capable of damaging or altering DNA directly, causing double-stranded (ds) breaks and the formation of cross-linked pyrimidine bases, such as thymidine dimers (TT), as particularly important byproducts. Carbon-centered radicals formed directly by ionizing radiation on the deoxyribose moiety of DNA are thought to be the precursors of strand breaks. Cells undergoing extensive irreparable DNA damage generally enter into apoptosis (programmed cell death), and surviving cells bear the hallmarks of radiation damage in the form of mutations, chromosomal abnormalities and genetic instability.

Rapidly dividing cells, such as the blood forming cells (hematopoietic) in bone marrow, germ cells in testes and ovary, mucosal lining cells of the gastrointestinal tract, airway, etc. are most susceptible to injury from ionizing radiation. Cells in the G_2

and mitotic phases of the cell cycle are the most likely to be damaged. In fact, it has been suggested that much of what is considered critical illness may involve oxygen radical ("oxyradical") pathophysiology. Oxyradical injury has been implicated in the pathogenesis of pulmonary oxygen toxicity, adult respiratory distress syndrome (ARDS), bronchopulmonary dysplasia, sepsis syndrome, and a variety of ischemia-reperfusion syndromes, including myocardial infarction, stroke, cardiopulmonary bypass, organ transplantation, necrotizing enterocolitis, acute renal tubular necrosis, and other diseases.

Radiation exposure from any source can be classified as acute (a single large exposure) or chronic (a series of small low-level, or continuous low-level exposures spread over time). Table 11-2 sets forth the radiation doses from selected sources. Radiation dosage is reported in millirem and radiation sickness generally results from an acute exposure of a sufficient dose, and presents with a characteristic set of symptoms that appear in an orderly fashion, including hair loss, weakness, vomiting, diarrhea, skin burns and bleeding from the gastrointestinal tract and mucous membranes.

TABLE 11-2

Source	Dose in Millirem
Television	<1/yr
Gamma Rays, Jet Cross Country	1
Mountain Vacation - 2 week	3
Atomic Test Fallout	5
U.S. Water, Food & Air (Average)	30/yr
Wood	50/yr
Concrete	50/yr
Brick	75/yr
Chest X-Ray	100
Cosmic Radiation (Sea Level)	40/yr (+1 millirem/100 ft elev.)
Natural Background San Francisco	120/yr
Natural Background Denver	50/yr
Atomic Energy Commission Limit for Workers	5,000/yr
Complete Dental X-Ray	5,000
Natural Background at Pocos de Caldras, Brazil	7,000/yr
Whole Body Diagnostic X-Ray	100,000
Cancer Therapy (localized)	500,000
Radiation Sickness-Nagasaki (single doses)	125,000
LD$_{50}$ Nagasaki & Hiroshima single dose	400,000-500,000

Genetic defects, sterility and cancers (particularly bone marrow cancer) often develop over time. A sufficiently large acute dose of ionizing radiation, for example 500,000 to over 1 million millirem (equivalent to 5-10 Gy), may kill a subject immediately. Doses in the hundreds of thousands of millirems may kill within 7 to 21 days from a condition called "acute radiation poisoning." An acute total body exposure of 125,000 millirem may cause radiation sickness. Localized doses such as are used in radiotherapy may not cause radiation sickness, but may result in the damage or death of exposed normal cells.

An acute total body radiation dose of 100,000-125,000 millirem (equivalent to 1 Gy) received in less than one week would result in observable physiologic effects such as skin burns or rashes, mucosal and GI bleeding, nausea, diarrhea and/or excessive fatigue. Longer term cytotoxic and genetic effects such as hematopoietic and immunocompetent cell destruction, hair loss (alopecia), gastrointestinal, and oral mucosal sloughing, venoocclusive disease of the liver and chronic vascular hyperplasia of cerebral vessels, cataracts, pneumonitis, skin changes, and an increased incidence of cancer may also manifest over time. Acute doses of less than 10,000 millirem (equivalent to 0.1 Gy) typically will not result in immediately observable biologic or physiologic effects, although long term cytotoxic or genetic effects may occur.

Chronic exposure is usually associated with delayed medical problems such as cancer and premature aging. Chronic radiation exposure is a low level

(i.e., 100-5,000 millirem) incremental or continuous radiation dose received over time. Examples
of chronic doses include a whole-body dose of
about 5,000 millirem per year, which is the dose
typically received by an adult human working at a
nuclear power plant. By contrast, the Atomic Energy Commission recommends that members of the
general public should receive no more than 100
millirem per year. Chronic doses may cause long-
term cytotoxic and genetic effects, for example
manifesting as an increased risk of a radiation-
induced cancer developing later in life.

Chronic doses of greater than 5,000 millirem per
year (0.05 Gy per year) may result in long-term
cytotoxic or genetic effects similar to those described for persons receiving acute doses. Some adverse cytotoxic or genetic effects may also occur at
chronic doses of significantly less than 5,000 millirem per year. For radiation protection purposes, it
is assumed that any dose above zero can increase
the risk of radiation-induced cancer (i.e., that there
is no threshold). Epidemiologic studies have found that the estimated lifetime risk of dying from
cancer is greater by about 0.04% per rem of radiation dose to the whole body.

A major source of (acute) exposure to ionizing radiation is the administration of human-derived therapeutic radiation in the treatment of cancer or other proliferative disorders. Subjects exposed to therapeutic doses of ionizing radiation typically receive between 0.1 and 2 Gy per treatment, and can receive as high as 5 Gy per treatment. Depending on the course of treatment prescribed by the treating physician, multiple doses may be received by a subject over the course of several weeks to several months.

Exposure to ionizing radiation from human-derived sources can also occur in the occupational setting. Occupational doses of ionizing radiation may be received by persons whose job involves exposure (or potential exposure) to radiation, for example in the nuclear power and nuclear weapons industries. Occupational exposure may also occur in rescue and emergency personnel called into deal with catastrophic events involving a nuclear reactor or radioactive materials. Other sources of occupational exposure may be from machine parts, plastics, solvents left over from the manufacture of radioactive medical products, smoke alarms, emergency signs, and other consumer goods. Exposure may also occur in military or civilian persons who serve on nuclear powered vessels, particularly those who tend the nuclear reactors, and those operating in areas contaminated by military uses of radioactive materials, including nuclear weapons fallout.

Mammals, including humans and other animals (such as livestock), may also be exposed to ionizing radiation of human derivation from the environment. The primary source of exposure to significant amounts of such environmental radiation is from nuclear power plant accidents, such as those at Three Mile Island, Chernobyl, Tokaimura, Fukushima etc. Environmental exposure to ionizing radiation may also result from nuclear weapons detonations (either experimental or during wartime), discharges of actinides from nuclear waste storage and processing and reprocessing of nuclear fuel, and from naturally occurring radioactive materials such as radon gas or uranium. There is also increasing concern that the use of ordnance containing depleted uranium results in low-level radioactive contamination of combat areas.

As noted above, for most mammals the bulk of their lifetime radiation exposure derives from naturally-occurring sources. Such sources include radioactive chemical elements dispersed throughout nature, such as the small amount of uranium that occurs naturally in granite. Small amounts of radioactive elements are found pervasively in the atmosphere, ground, and water, to lesser and greater degrees depending upon location. Other significant naturally-occurring sources derive from outer space: the sun and the cosmos. Ultra-violet radiation emitted by the sun may be particularly hazardous as relatively strong doses may be acquired accidentally throughout much of the world. Cosmic radiation, x-ray, and gamma radiation exposure is of particular risk to those living or working at high altitudes. Commercial and military flight personnel, including astronauts, are particularly susceptible to such radiation owing to the relatively long periods they spend at high-altitudes.

While anti-radiation suits or other protective gear may be effective at reducing radiation exposure, such gear is expensive, unwieldy, and generally not available to public. Moreover, radioprotective gear will not protect normal tissue adjacent a tumor from stray radiation exposure during radiotherapy. What is needed, therefore, is a practical way to protect subjects who are scheduled to incur, or are at risk for incurring, exposure to ionizing radiation. In the context of therapeutic irradiation, it is desirable to enhance protection of normal cells while causing tumor cells to remain vulnerable to the detrimental effects of the radiation. Furthermore, it will be appropriate to provide systemic protection from anticipated or inadvertent total body irradiation, such as may occur with occupational or environmental exposures, or with certain therapeutic techniques.

Pharmaceutical radioprotectants offer a cost-efficient, effective and easily available alternative to radioprotective gear. However, previous attempts at radioprotection of normal cells with pharmaceutical compositions have not been entirely successful. For example, cytokines directed at mobilizing the peripheral blood progenitor cells confer a myeloprotective effect when given prior to radiation, but do not confer systemic protection. Other chemical radioprotectors administered alone or in combination with biologic response modifiers have shown minor protective effects in mice, but application of these compounds to large mammals was less successful, and it was questioned whether chemical radioprotection was of any value.

Urgency for Radiation Protection

In today's heightened nuclear threat from terrorists and/or rogue nations as well as accidents in nuclear power-plant reactors (Fukushima Daiichi in Japan following an earthquake and tsunami in March 2011), there is an increased need to have safe and effective means to protect the nuclear-reactor workers and the population at large from the health hazards of ionizing radiation exposures. The United States Department of Energy (DOE) reports that "an unfilled dream of civil and military officials concerned with this issue is to have a globally effective pharmacologic, i.e. the magic radioprotective pill. This pill could be taken orally without any undue side effects prior to or after a suspected nuclear/radiological event in order to provide the individual full bodily protection against early arising acute injury and late arising pathologies[1]." Thus, a "radioprotective pill" is of urgent and vital national security interest.

The DOE report further states:

"…Currently a full range of R&D strategies are being employed in the hunt for new safe and effective radioprotectants including: a) large scale screening of newly identified chemical classes or natural products; b) reformulating or restructuring

---

[1] United States Department of Energy Report of July 13, 2005 on Inositol and Other Radioprotective Agents Workshop, Cambridge. Massachusetts.

older protectants with proven efficacies to reduce unwanted toxicities; c) using **_nutraceuticals_** [bold and italics added] that are only moderately protective but that are essentially non-toxic and exceedingly well tolerated; d) using low dose combinations of potentially toxic (at high drug doses) but efficacious agents that cytoprotect through different routes in hopes of fostering radioprotective synergy; and e) accepting lower drug efficacy in lieu of non-toxicity, banking on the protection afforded by the drug can be leveraged by post-exposure therapies...Inositol hexaphosphate, IP-6, and its analogs are entering testing as drugs. One of the challenges is to cover phosphates with protecting groups, to facilitate passage of the molecule into the cell. (DOE report of July 13, 2005)." Implied is the notion that IP_6 and its derivatives, including pyrophosphates, and/or inositol may currently be ineffective as radioprotectants!

Efforts to find radio-modifiers, such as radio-protectors and radio-sensitizers in the past have focused on hypoxic cell sensitizers such as metranidazole and misonidazole. Radioprotectors have received much less attention than radio-sensitizers at the clinical level. The nuclear era spawned considerable effort in the development of radioprotectors with more than 4,000 compounds being synthesized and tested at the Walter Reed Army Institute of Research in the USA in the 1960's. With the exception of a compound known as WR2727, none of those compounds has proven useful in either the military or industrial contexts or for cancer radiotherapy.

IP₆ + Inositol to the Rescue

IP₆ and inositol protect human cells against radiation damage in the laboratory (*in vitro*) in various ways. For example, while irradiation caused increased cell death (loss of cell attachment, apoptosis and necrosis) IP₆ and inositol treatment prevented cell death, *in vitro*. *In vivo* (in laboratory mice) IP₆ significantly reduced the incidence and multiplicity of UV-induced skin tumors in mice (Kolappaswamy *et al* 2009).

In one of our *in vitro* experiments, human keratinocyte HaCaT cells were exposed to UVB 30 mJ/cm2 (2 minutes 10 seconds); non-exposed cells served as control. The cells were then treated with IP₆, Inositol, IP₆+Inositol, and untreated (control) and placed in the incubator for 18 hours. The cells that remained attached to the wells are live (protected from UVB damage); the number of attached cells is measured by dissolving them in acetic acid and measuring the optical absorbance of the solution (please see Figure 11-1).

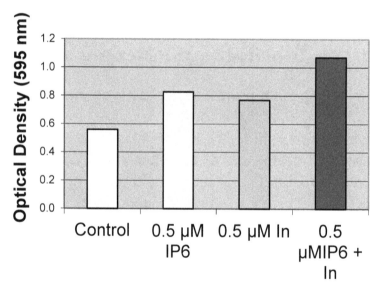

Figure 11-1: Following UVB exposure, as signs of cellular injury and death, the control untreated cells show less attachment to the plate as opposed to those treated with Na-IP₆, Inositol (In) and IP₆ + Inositol. Please note that the cells treated with 1:1 molar ratio of IP₆ and Inositol showed the best attachment, hence best protected.

In the *in vivo* experiment, mice were irradiated 3 times a week, initially with 1.5 kJ/m² dose and escalating weekly by 1.5 kJ/m² to a final dose of 7.5 kJ/m²; each session lasted approximately 10 min for 23 weeks. Animals were fed with AIN-76A diet that does not contain IP₆. About 100 mg of IP₆ ± Inositol was applied on the dorsal surface topically in skin cream as 4% K-IP₆, 1% inositol, 4% K-IP₆ + 1% inositol. An additional group received IP₆+inositol at 1:1 molar ratio in drinking water to see if orally administered IP₆+ inositol would provide similar protection.

Table 11-3 shows that animals that were treated with IP₆ in skin cream had no tumors as opposed to the cream without IP₆; IP₆+inositol in skin cream showed a 60% reduction in tumors and even more interestingly animals who received IP₆+ inositol in drinking water had a 78.6% reduction in UVB-induced skin tumor incidence.

And that's not all. A report in the journal *Radiation Protection Dosimetry* (2007) by Dr. D. Cebrian and colleagues from the Radiobiology Laboratory of the Department of Environment,

Table 11-3

Experimental Groups (n=15 in each group)	Percentage of Mice with Tumors
Vehicle (cream) + UVB	71.4
K-IP₆ (4% in cream) + UVB	0
Inositol (1% in cream) + UVB	58.3
K-IP₆ + Inositol (4% + 1% in cream) + UVB	28.6
Na-IP₆ 2% in drinking water + UVB	15.3

CIEMAT, Madrid, Spain, show "strong affinity of inositol hexaphosphate (IP₆) for uranium, suggesting that it could be an effective chelating agent for uranium in vivo." Given the paucity of available protectants let alone the low effectiveness and/or side-effects, the safety of IP₆ makes it a superior candidate.

The preceding strongly suggest that IP₆+inositol could help protect us from various forms of radiation damage such as UV from sun-exposure, radiation therapy, cosmic radiation, accidental or induced nuclear blasts etc. The methods of administration could be either in the form of skin cream and/or orally.

CHAPTER 12

IP$_6$+INOSITOL & DIABETES MELLITUS

Diabetes, a Global Epidemic

Diabetes Mellitus (DM) is a chronic condition that afflicts an estimated 221 million or more people worldwide (more than 3% of the world population) in 2010. It is as a result of either **insufficient secretion of insulin** from the pancreas or when the **body cannot effectively use the insulin** it produces, resulting in hyperglycemia (increased blood sugar level).

The World Health Organization (WHO) estimates that the number of diabetics (>180 million) is likely to more than double by the year 2030. WHO also estimated that in 2005, approximately 1.1 million people died from diabetes worldwide. Almost 80% of diabetes deaths occur in low and middle-income countries. There are 20.8 million adults and children in the United States, or 7% of the population, who have diabetes; unfortunately, over one-third of whom (6.2 million people) are unaware that they have the disease.

Almost half of diabetes deaths occur in people under the age of 70 years; 55% of deaths due to diabetes are in women. WHO projects that deaths due to diabetes will increase by more than 50% in the next 10 years unless means are adopted to control the disease. Worse, deaths due to diabetes are estimated to increase by over 80% in upper-middle income countries between 2006 and 2015. Thus, there is an urgent need to prevent and control this global scourge.

There are two basic forms of diabetes: Type 1: people with this type of diabetes produce very little or no insulin. Type 2: people with this type of diabetes cannot use insulin effectively. Most people with diabetes have type 2. A third type of diabetes, gestational diabetes mellitus (GDM), develops during some cases of pregnancy but usually disappears after pregnancy.

Aside from the acute complications of diabetes, the late complications of diabetes mellitus affect multiple organ systems and are the chief causes of morbidity and mortality. The risks of the late complications vary markedly amongst individuals but are generally dependent on the duration of the disease – the longer the disease, the higher are the risks. These include: diabetic retinopathy, neuropathy, kidney disease, heart disease, stroke and peripheral vascular disease.

Diabetic retinopathy is an important cause of blindness; after 15 years of diabetes, approximately 2% of people become blind, and about 10% develop severe visual impairment. Diabetic neuropathy affects up to 50% of people. Combined with reduced blood flow (diabetic peripheral vascular disease), neuropathy in the feet increases the chance of foot ulcers and eventual limb amputation. And it increases the risk of heart disease and stroke; about 50% of people with diabetes die of cardiovascular disease - heart disease and stroke. In addition, people with diabetes suffer from cataract, weakened immune response – frequent bouts of infections; diabetic mothers have higher risks of miscarriages and birth-defects in off-springs (diabetic embryopathy). As if these are not grim enough, the overall risk of dying among people with diabetes is at least double the risk of their peers without it.

What causes the complications? The inability to utilize glucose by the cells results in excessive glucose in blood and diminished glucose available for energy metabolism by the cells dependent on this fuel. On one hand the excessive glucose binds with the protein in the blood (glycosylated hemoglobin HbA$_{1c}$ as an example, used to monitor the disease) and tissues. The latter causes irreversible formation of advanced glycosylated end products (AGE) which accumulate over the life-time of the vessel wall. AGE cross-link peptides of some proteins such as collagen, induce lipid oxidation, inactivate nitric oxide, bind nucleic acids etc. These are considered to be fundamental to the vascular, renal and other complications.

The cellular metabolism is also affected on the other hand. The vast majority of cells dependent on insulin for taking up glucose suffer from a deficiency of intracellular inositol level, which in turn affects the signal transduction pathways within the cell. And those cells that are not dependent on insulin suffer from intracellular hyperglycemia leading to increased intracellular sorbitol with resultant cell injury. These mechanisms are considered to be at play in diabetic neuropathy, retinopathy, renal vascular disease, etc.

Studies suggest that oxidative damage is also responsible for some of the complications such as cataract and embryopathy.

How can IP$_6$+Inositol help?

Role of IP$_6$:

During the secretion of insulin by the pancreatic β cells, the hormone is extruded from the cell by a process called exocytosis. Essentially it is like scooping up the hormone with a part of the cell membrane and closing it up in the manner of a purse string, taking it to the cell surface, opening it up and extruding it. Glucose is the signal that tells the β cells when to secrete insulin. In human Type II diabetes (the vast majority), loss of this glucose-stimulated insulin exocytosis from the pancreatic β cells is an early pathogenetic event.

Studies done in Karolinska Institute in Stockholm showed that the concentration of IP$_6$ within the pancreatic β cells transiently increases upon glucose stimulation. It happens in a dose-dependent manner with differential inhibition of the enzyme ser/thr protein phosphatases. Interestingly, none of the oral hypoglycemic sulfonylureas tested by Lehtihet *et al* (2004) affected protein phosphatase-1 or -2A activity at clinically relevant concentrations in these cells. Thus, the authors conclude:

"….an increase in cellular phosphorylation state, through inhibition of protein dephosphorylation by InsP₆ [IP₆] may be a novel regulatory mechanism linking glucose-stimulated polyphosphoinositide formation to insulin exocytosis in insulin-secreting cells."

Translated in plain English: IP$_6$ is needed for insulin secretion!

Now, combine that with the paper by Dr. Lowell Dilworth and colleagues in Kingston, Jamaica, published in the March 2005 issue of the *West Indian Medical Journal* volume 56: pages 102-106: They demonstrated that IP$_6$ supplementation in diet caused a lowering of blood glucose level in experimental rats.

That was in rats. C57BL/6N mice are widely used for the investigation of the pathophysiology of impaired glucose tolerance and Type 2 diabetes to look for new therapeutics. Dr. Soo Mi Kim and colleagues from the Kyungpook National University in Daegu, Republic of Korea investigated the effect of IP₆ on the glucose metabolizing enzymes in these mice given a high-fat diet. They report in the July 2010 issue of the *Journal of Clinical Biochemistry & Nutrition* that **IP₆ treated mice showed a marked decrease in blood glucose level, higher glucokinase and glucose-6-phosphatase activity, higher hepatic glycogen and considerably lower bodyweight than control mice**.

Recently, IP₆ has been found to be useful in treatment of diabetes from a different angle: Owing to the inconvenience of daily injection of insulin, the quest for finding alternative methods has been going on. Dr. Lee and colleagues at Yonsei University, Seoul, Korea, have used IP₆ as a crosslinking agent for encapsulation of insulin in a chitosan matrix for oral delivery. IP₆-chitosan capsules were compared with tripolyphosphate (TPP)-chitosan capsules for stable oral delivery of insulin. During a 2 h incubation in simulated gastric fluid, IP$_6$-chitosan capsules showed better stability than TPP-chitosan capsules. IP$_6$-chitosan capsules released less than 60% of their encapsulated insulin after 24 h incubation in simulated gastrointestinal fluids; in contrast, TPP-chitosan capsules released virtually the entire insulin content within 12 h. When studied *in vivo* using diabetic mice IP$_6$-chitosan capsules significantly decreased blood glucose levels while TPP-chitosan capsules caused a lesser reduction. The relative pharmacological bioactivity of IP$_6$-chitosan capsules was 6.4% while that of TPP-chitosan capsules was 1.1%. "PA [IP$_6$]-chitosan capsules appeared to have good potential for use in oral delivery of insulin for sustained control of the blood glucose level" conclude the authors (Lee *et al* 2011).

It would be interesting to know what, if any, the contribution of IP$_6$ was in lowering the blood glucose level.

Inositol:

I had already referred to the landmark paper by Nascimento *et al* in January 2006 entitled: "Inositols prevent and reverse endothelial dysfunction in diabetic rat and rabbit vasculature metabolically and by scavenging superoxide." the title says it all!

The endothelial cells that form the inner linings of blood vessels are damaged in diabetes; this is a first step in the process of atherosclerosis. The study results strongly suggest that cardiovascular complications of diabetes could potentially be prevented if not reversed by inositol. The researchers also found that inositols (there are a few different isomers of inositol) decreased both the elevated blood sugar and triglyceride levels of the test animals.

Inositol enhanced the action of nitrous oxide and acted as a potent antioxidant as well. And you also know that IP_6 is also a very potent antioxidant. This takes us to the next issue: the other complications of diabetes related to oxidative damage such as cataract, diabetic embryopathy, etc. As potent antioxidants IP_6+inositol should inhibit cataract formation.

Additional Complications of DM

Congenital malformations involving the heart and the nervous system occur more often in children born to diabetic mothers. The incidence of an abnormality in the embryo (embryopathy) in diabetic mothers is 4 to 5 times higher than average. Prof.

E. Albert Reece, then at Temple University in Philadelphia, and currently our Dean of the Faculty of Medicine at the University of Maryland in Baltimore, and his team found that the inositol levels in the embryonic tissues were significantly lower than the control. They showed that by adding inositol to the diet of the diabetic mothers (rats in these experiments) they could significantly reduce the incidence of neural tube defects when compared to the diabetic rats not receiving inositol supplementation. On one hand while their study suggests that inositol deficiency may play a very important role in diabetic embryopathy, inositol supplementation could ameliorate the problem on the other. They propose that excessive oxidation by oxygen free radicals and changes in the inositol level in the embryo to be the pathogenetic mechanism for diabetic embryopathy (Zhao & Reece 2005). Dean Reece and his team of investigators proved that to be case; although they did not use IP$_6$, they however gave inositol supplementation and other antioxidants to decrease the malformation rates.

"The experimental use of several different compounds, such as arachidonic acid, myo-inositol, and antioxidants, offer significant promise for the future in possibly serving as a pharmaco-

logical prophylaxis against diabetic embryopathy." [EA Reece & UJ Eriksson. Obstetrics and Gynecology Clinics of North America volume 23: pages 29-45, March 1996].

Human Study

We have learnt about the experiments in mice and rats; what about us humans and how does diet (and fiber) fit in all these? LN Panlasigui and LU Thompson from the University of Philippines in Quezon City compared the blood glucose lowering effect of milled-rice versus brown rice (which has its bran and therefore high levels of IP_6 and inositol) in 10 healthy and 9 Type II diabetic volunteers. They report in the *International Journal of Food Sciences and Nutrition* (May-June issue 2006, volume 57: pages 151-158) a blood glucose lowering effect of brown rice.

"The effect was partly due to the higher amounts of phytic acid [IP₆], polyphenols, dietary fiber and oil in brown compared to milled rice..." concluded the authors.

This goes back to the issues we discussed early on in the book about mothers' wisdom: eat a healthy diet. But if you need extra protection, there is IP$_6$+ inositol!

To summarize, IP$_6$ and inositol independently may help in diabetes by i) stimulating insulin secretion by the pancreatic β cells (IP$_6$) and by ii) reducing the oxidative damage to the cells and tissues inflicted through AGE; both IP$_6$ and inositol can prevent that as antioxidants. iii) Both IP$_6$ and inositol could replenish the low intracellular inositol levels as neither of them requires insulin to gain entry into the cell; once inside the cells, IP$_6$ can shed its phosphates and enter into the intracellular inositol-inositol phosphate pool. Thus IP$_6$+ inositol is the perfect combination!

CHAPTER 13

ATHEROSCLEROTIC CARDIOVASCULAR DISEASE

Atherosclerosis means hardening of arteries, and is also believed to have been prevalent since the ancient Egypt [recall, cancer too was described by the ancient Egyptian physician Imhotep around 2625 B.C.E.]. It is characterized by *atheroma* or fibrofatty plaques in the innermost layer (intima) of the arteries. These atheromas protrude into the lumen thereby narrowing the luminal space, and weaken the media. The so diseased artery can be calcified, a fact noted as early as the sixteenth century as "degeneration of arteries into bone" (Gregory *et al* 2009).

While atherosclerosis is extremely common in Europe and North America, it is much less prevalent in Africa, Asia, and South and Central America. Atherosclerosis is the cause of ischemic heart disease (atherosclerotic cardiovascular disease ASCVD) which causes morbidity and mortality; the United States has one of the highest rates. Japan on the other hand, has a fifth the mortality rate from heart attack than that of USA. However, the rate is increasing in Japan and Japanese who migrate to USA and adopt the life-style and dietary habit customs of their adopted home become more susceptible. This is true not just for atherosclerotic cardiovascular diseases, but also for cancers, especially that of the colon and rectum. This observation points to the role of environmental risk factors aside from the genetic predispositions, to pathogenesis of atherosclerosis. Diet, physical activity, cigarette smoking, diabetes, high blood pressure, are clearly very important in predisposing to ASCVD.

Atheroma Formation

The atheromatous plaque consists of a focally rai-
sed plaque within the intima[1] with a core of lipid
(mostly composed of cholesterol or cholesterol
esters) covered with a fibrous cap. Almost invariably, atheromas become calcified as the condition
progresses; this is one of the commonest complications of atherosclerosis rendering the artery like
pipe stem with eggshell brittleness. As you can
imagine, this makes the affected artery susceptible
to more complications. Thus affected artery may
undergo ulceration or even rupture, liberating the
debris from the atheroma to the blood which may
travel to distant sites (emboli) and cause damage
therein. There could also be hemorrhage within the
plaque acutely compromising the lumen of the
vessel. And then, the thus damaged plaque could
be the seat of thrombosis with partial or total obstruction of the lumen resulting in infarction of the
organ (e.g. heart attack).

---

[1] The innermost of the three layers of the artery, the others
are media (*tunica media*) – in the middle and the adventitia
(*tunica adventitia*).

Let's first look at how atherosclerosis forms and how IP_6 can affect the very genesis of atherosclerosis.

Insofar as the genesis of atherosclerosis is concerned, historically there have been two major schools of thoughts, each emphasizing either cellular proliferation in the intima or thrombosis in the arterial wall. The view now-a-days considers atherosclerosis to be a chronic inflammatory response of the arterial wall secondary to an injury to the endothelial cells lining the inner surface (lumen) of the arteries. While endothelial injury has produced atheroma experimentally, early human lesions of atheroma begin at sites that show no evidence of injury, at least morphologically. That may point to other forms of injury or disruption of normalcy such as increased endothelial permeability, increased adhesion of leukocytes to the endothelium etc.

The adhesion of leukocytes to the endothelium is dependent on binding of the complementary adhesion molecules on the leukocytes and the endothelial cells; certain chemicals influence this binding ability by modulating the surface expression of these adhesion molecules or by modifying their avidity. There are several groups of adhesion molecules: the selectins, immunoglobulins, integrins, etc. Selectins are composed of three different types, depending on their location in the cell types: E-selectin (confined to endothelial cells), L-selectin in leukocytes hence "L" and P-selectin present in platelets, hence "P" (but also present in endothe-lium). Selectins bind through their lectin domain to sialylated forms of carbohydrate such as sialy-lated Lewis X.

Why am I going into these details, and what does IP₆ has to do with all this? It turns out that IP₆ in-hibits the binding of L- and P-selectin to sialyl Lewis X (Cecconi *et al.*, 1994). M. Shimazawa *et al* from Hamamatsu University School of Medi-cine in Japan (European Journal of Pharmacology 2005 Sep 27; 520:156-63) investigated the role of leukocytes in the pathogenesis of atherosclerosis. They asked the question: would neutrophil accu-mulation participate in the development of inti-mal hyperplasia after endothelial injury in mice? They also wanted to test whether IP₆ which inhi-bits the binding of L- and P-selectin to sialyl Lewis X could inhibit the development of intimal hyper-plasia. Endothelial injury was induced in the femo-ral artery (70 mice) *via* the photochemical reaction between systemically injected Rose Bengal and transillumination with green light (wavelength: 540 nm). At 3 days after injury, scanning electron microscopy showed an increase in the number of leukocytes adhering to the injury site. They treated the mice with antibody to produce neutropenia (reduced number of neutrophils) that resulted in a significant decrease in the intimal area in the injured vessel compared to the control group. In another experiment, treatment with IP$_6$ produced a significant decrease in the intimal area. Their data suggest that neutrophil accumulation on the injured vessels may contribute to initiation and development of intimal hyperplasia and that either neutropenia or IP$_6$ inhibit that process. Since induction of neutropenia is not an option [owing to the risk of infection], IP$_6$ is a better alternative!

Role of Platelets

Platelets become activated at the site of vascular injury. While on one hand, platelet activation at a site of damage of a blood vessel to form a clot is essential for arresting the bleeding, excessive platelet activation on the other hand can result in the unwarranted formation of arterial thrombi, the consequence of which is precipitating acute myocardial infarction, or stroke. The three-main events in thrombus formation are that a) the platelets must adhere to the site of injury (platelet adhesion), b) they must aggregate with each other, and finally c) they have to be activated – main trigger being damaged endothelium; human platelets contain matrix metalloproteinase 2 (MMP-2) and release it upon activation; active MMP-2 amplifies the platelet aggregation response and plays a critical role in thrombus formation. Therefore, adhesion of platelets to the inner layer of the artery, their aggregation and finally activation are the earliest events in the formation of thrombus and atherosclerosis. Thus, it is not surprising that a lot of effort to reduce atherosclerotic cardiovascular diseases is directed towards blocking or slowing down some of these steps. The antiplatelet therapy (aspirin is the most familiar one) aims to decrease the activity of circulating platelets and block the secretion of platelet granules containing the platelet-derived thrombotic factors. And the most clinically relevant test for monitoring the state of platelet health insofar as thrombogenic potential is platelet aggregation assay.

My colleagues Drs. Vucenik, Podczasy and I looked at the ability of IP₆ to inhibit human platelet aggregation from 10 healthy volunteers. The platelets were activated by known activators – ADP, collagen and thrombin, in the presence or absence of IP_6. Figure 13-1 shows that IP_6 significantly ($p<0.0001$) inhibited platelet aggregation in a dose-dependent manner; the higher the dose of IP_6 the stronger was the inhibition. Note the very high statistical significance.

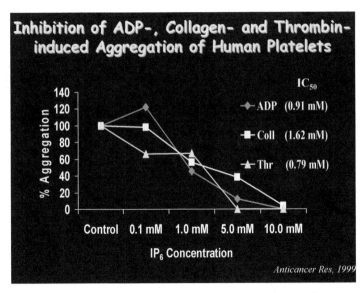

Figure 13-1: Increased concentration of IP_6 increasingly inhibits abnormal platelet aggregation.

IP_6 also significantly reduced the release of ATP from the granules ($p=0.00247$ for ADP, $p=0.0074$ for collagen and $p=0.0069$ for thrombin). Thus, it is quite plausible that IP_6 may help prevent atherosclerotic cardiovascular diseases through this mechanism.

Calcification of Atherosclerotic Plaques

As mentioned earlier, one of the complications of atherosclerosis is calcification of the plaques which render the arteries susceptible to thrombosis, rupture etc. Patients with a high degree of calcification of coronary arteries are at increased risk for these coronary artery events. Calcification of the arteries and heart valves is also age-related, with increased age there is increased calcification, the latter contributing to heart failure as well.

Enter Prof. Grases [again, and again...!]. His lab evaluated the effect of IP_6 on cardiovascular calcification in rats during aging. Ten weeks old were fed with either a balanced diet containing IP_6, or a purified diet that had no detectable IP_6. or purified diet + IP_6 and purified diet with inositol. At 76 weeks of age all rats were sacrificed, and the aortas, hearts, kidneys, livers and femurs were removed for chemical analysis. The most significant result was the difference in the calcium content of the aorta. IP$_6$-treated rats had significantly lower levels of calcium in the aorta compared to rats fed diet without IP$_6$, thus demonstrating that IP$_6$ treatment significantly reduces age-related calcification of the aorta.

And that's not all. Prof. Grases further extended his investigation to other tissues besides the aorta. In another experiment, his lab pretreated rats with IP$_6$ for 16 days [as I had done in the cancer prevention study; recall the pre-initiation experiment] induced abnormal calcification in rats by giving them intramuscular injection of high doses of Vitamin D and oral nicotine (Grases *et al* 2006). After 60 hours of this calcinosis treatment, all of the rats not treated with IP$_6$ died. A highly significant increase in the calcium content in the aorta and heart muscle was observed in the control IP$_6$ non-treated rats (21 ± 1 mg calcium/g dry aorta tissue, 10 ± 1 mg calcium/g dry heart tissue) when compared with controls (1.3 ± 0.1 mg calcium/g dry aorta tissue, 0.023 ± 0.004 mg calcium/g heart dry tissue). Compared to the IP$_6$ *non*-treated rats, the IP$_6$-treated animals had much lower calcium content not just in the aorta (0.9 ± 0.2 mg calcium/g dry aorta, about same as the healthy control) but also in the heart (0.30± 0.03 mg calcium/g dry heart tissue)!

Let's now move on to the next step in the havoc atherosclerosis plays and how IP$_6$ can be relevant in here as well.

Heart Attack

Occlusion of the artery feeding a tissue or organ causes ischemic injury as in heart attack (myocardial infarction) from coronary artery blockage, or stroke following carotid artery obstruction. The cells in the affected area are deprived of oxygen, irreversibly injured and die. The infarcted tissue however does not show a uniform picture – areas of dead cells are interspersed with still viable ones. Patients with acute myocardial infarction are at a risk of heart failure, irregular heart beat (arrthymia) and death. Thus, early restoration of the blood supply that has been cut-off from the heart is not only desirable but also essential for salvaging the heart. Paradoxically, this restoration or reperfusion can exacerbate myocardial damage – a process called reperfusion injury; depending on the duration and severity of the ischemic event, a variable number of cells die *after* the blood flow resumes!

One of the mechanisms responsible for this reperfusion injury is the reactive oxygen species (ROS). Furthermore, oxygen-derived free radicals reduce myocardial contractility and ventricular function, rendering the heart prone to failure.

Pre-treatment with some antioxidants, such as pyrrolidine dithiocarbamate (PDTC) or N-acetylcysteine, as well as some vitamins with recognized antioxidant properties, namely ascorbic acid (vitamin C), all-trans Retinoic Acid (atRA) and α-tocopherol (vitamin E) can suppress oxidative stress-induced tissue factor expression in human coronary artery endothelial cells (De Rosa *et al* 2010).

Since the chelation of Fe^{3+} by iron-chealtors such as deferoxamine mesylate reduced myocardial reperfusion injury, Dr. Parinam Rao and colleagues at the Long Island Jewish Medical Center and Albert Einstein College of Medicine in New York, and the University of Connecticut College of Medicine in Farmington investigated whether IP$_6$ by virtue of its antioxidant property would also protect the heart from reperfusion injury. Their study was further motivated by the fact that not only IP$_6$ is a natural antioxidant, but IP$_6$ has the "unique ability to remove O_2 without generating oxyradicals," thereby IP_6 could reduce free radical-mediated myocardial damage. (Rao *et al* 1991).

IP_6 was injected intravenously to rats in three different dose levels 30 minutes before the hearts were removed from the body. The minimum dose was 15 mg/kg (corresponding to 1.05 g for a 70-kg human), maximum dose of 150 mg/kg body weight corresponding to 10.5g for a 70-kg human and an intermediate dose of 75 mg/kg (5.25 g for a 70-kg human). The control group received saline solution only. Global ischemia was induced in isolated hearts for 30 minutes, followed by another 30 minutes of reperfusion. Not unexpectedly reperfusion was associated with increased creatine kinase release[2] and reduced coronary artery flow. As evidenced by reduced left ventricular developed pressure and the first derivative of left ventricular pressure, the ventricular function also recovered poorly. IP_6 did not alter left ventricular contractility *before* ischemia. However after 30 minutes of reperfusion following the ischemic insult, only the hearts from animals in the intermediate- and high-dose IP_6-treatment group (equivalent to 5.25 and 10.5 g IP_6 for a 70 kg human), but not the low dose-group showed better recovery of left ventri-

---

[2] Release of creatine kinase is a sensitive indicator of myocardial infarction.

cular developed pressure and the first derivative of left ventricular pressure compared to the control untreated group; the results were statistically significant at $p<0.05$. Insofar as coronary artery flow was concerned, IP_6 did not increase the coronary artery flow significantly ($p>0.05$). However, during the re-perfusion period, hearts from IP_6-treated rats showed a higher recovery of coronary artery flow as compared to the untreated saline controls.

The scientists examined free radical formation and quenching by producing •OH by xanthine oxidase on hypoxanthine in the presence of $FeCl_3$. A specific •OH scavenger dimethylsulfoxide decreased •OH signal. The formation of •OH in the hearts was quantitated by measuring •OH salicylate product 2,3- and 2,5-dihydroxybenzoic acid with high pressure liquid chromatography coupled with an electrochemical detector. The formation of •OH was significantly ($p<0.05$) reduced in the hearts of animals receiving the intermediate and high dose of IP_6. "*These results suggest potential use of this antioxidant [IP₆] in salvaging the heart from ischemic and reperfusion injury.*" concluded the authors.

CHAPTER 14

BONE, STONE & TOOTH

Osteoporosis

Osteoporosis represents a group of diseases characterized by reduced bone mass per unit of bone volume resulting in weak and fragile bone with increased risks of fractures of hip, wrist and spine. In the United States, nearly 10 million people already have osteoporosis. Another 18 million people have low bone mass that places them at an increased risk for developing osteoporosis.

Eighty percent of those with osteoporosis are women. Of people older than 50 years, 1 in 2 women and 1 in 8 men are predicted to have an osteoporosis-related fracture in their lifetime; this is the commonest bone disease a physician sees in his/her practice.

There are many risk factors for osteoporosis, most notable are old-age, estrogen deficiency, genetic predisposition, nutritional factors etc. While bone may appear deceptively lifeless, it *is* a living tissue, for it is being continually broken down by cells called osteoclasts, and at the same time it is being reconstructed by cells called osteoblasts. It is the balance between these cells that determines whether we gain or lose bone. Bis-phosphonates, a group of *synthetic* polyphosphates are the most common medications prescribed for osteoporosis treatment and they include Fosamax, Actonel, Boniva, Reclast etc. While in general they are safe, as in almost all drugs, they too are not without complications. In contrast to bisphosphonates, as you have gathered by now, IP$_6$ is a natural compound that is also a polyphosphate (6 phosphate groups!). Thus, Prof. Félix Grases at the University of Balearic Islands and his colleagues have investigated the role of IP$_6$ in osteoporosis. As a first step, they setout to look for any correlation between dietary IP_6 and osteoporosis.

So, in an epidemiological study they (López-González *et al* 2008) have investigated the relationship between the risk of osteoporosis and dietary IP_6 consumption. Bone mineral density was determined in about 2,000 volunteers by means of dual radiological absorptiometry in the calcaneus or the lumbar column and the neck of the femur. Dietary information related to IP_6 consumption was acquired by questionnaires conducted on two different occasions. The authors found that the bone mineral density increased with increasing dietary IP_6 consumption. Multivariate linear regression analysis indicated that body weight and low IP_6 consumption were the risk factors with greatest influence on bone mineral density. The authors conclude:

"Phytate [IP₆] consumption had a protective effect against osteoporosis, suggesting that low phytate [IP₆] consumption should be considered an osteoporosis risk factor."

The investigators further proved it experimentally by using ovariectomized rats, a good model for post-menopausal osteoporosis as it causes estrogen deficiency (F Grases *Medicinal Food* 2009).

Ovariectomized rats were fed standard chow with or without Ca-Mg-IP$_6$ for 12 weeks following which their femoral and vertebral bones were carefully studied. Urinary deoxypyridinoline, a marker for bone resorption and serum osteocalcin (a marker for bone formation) were measured. The animals treated with IP$_6$ had higher calcium and phosphorous contents in bone and bone mineral density than the untreated control animals. Not unexpectedly, the bone resorption marker deoxy-pyridinoline was higher in the urine of animals that did not receive IP$_6$. Clearly, their study shows a great potential for the use of IP$_6$ in the prevention and treatment of osteoporosis.

This intriguing research also asked the question whether Ca-Mg-IP$_6$ would protect against predni-sone-induced bone loss. Even at very high doses of prednisone, the animals with IP$_6$ in their food had very little bone loss as compared to the ani-mals that did not receive IP$_6$. Calcium or magne-sium alone does not provide such protection. Ba-sed on the remarkable bone protective affects found to date, clinical trials are now underway to see whether Ca-Mg-IP$_6$ will protect people to the same extent as it does animals.

Experiments in my lab with sodium-IP_6 found stimulation of the bone building cells and at the same time inhibition of the bone resorbing cells *in vitro*. It is important to note that the affect was achieved with sodium-IP_6 and not Ca-Mg-IP_6 and therefore the changes were not due to calcium or magnesium. Rather it is my humble opinion that this bone-protective quality was due to IP_6 itself. Even more intriguing is the fact that emerging data show a strong interaction between the osteoblasts and osteoclasts in one hand and their effect *via* osteocalcin on the pancreatic β cells hence insulin secretion and bodyweight etc. on the other (Karsenty & Ferron 2012). Further research will unravel the additional mechanisms of IP_6's many functions.

Calcium: The Good, the Bad and the Ugly!

There are many roles of calcium in the body - intracellular communication (signal transduction), electrolyte balance and electrical conductivity, bone formation etc, functions vital to our survival. An acutely decreased serum calcium level can result in life-threatening cardiac arrhythmias or laryngeal spasm, whereas calcium deficiency over an extended period results in bone diseases. And excess calcium is not healthy either.

Cardiovascular Calcification

When there is abnormal deposition of calcium salts, together with a small amount of iron, magnesium and other mineral salts, in the tissue, it is called pathologic calcification. When the deposition takes place locally in diseased or dead tissue or cells, it is called **dystrophic calcification**. In disorders of calcium metabolism and hormone imbalances, calcification may take place in otherwise healthy normal tissue; this is called **metastatic calcification**. Of course, if the serum calcium level is already high, any damage, degeneration or necrosis will enhance pathological calcification.

Common examples of dystrophic calcification are those in our arteries as in advanced atherosclerosis. Prof. Grases has been working on the issue of pathological calcification and means to prevent it particularly by IP₆. He and his colleagues induced calcific atherosclerosis in rats by Vitamin D and nicotine and treated them with standard cream with or without IP₆. They observed a highly significant increase in the calcium content of aorta and heart tissue in the non-IP$_6$ treated rats (21 ± 1 mg calcium/g in aorta and 10 ± 1 mg calcium/g in heart) as compared to only 1.3 ± 0.1 mg and 0.023 ± 0.004 mg in the control group respectively. When they measured the calcium content in the IP$_6$-treated rat aorta and heart tissue, the amounts they found were similar, if not even lower than the control: 0.9 ± 0.2 mg calcium/g in aorta and 0.30 ± 0.03 mg calcium/g in the heart. They conclude:

"Only InsP6 non-treated rats displayed important mineral deposits in aorta and heart. These findings are consistent with the action of InsP6 [IP$_6$], as an inhibitor of calcification of cardiovascular system."

Calcinosis cutis

Calcinosis cutis is another example of pathologic calcification of the skin, seen in a variety of conditions such as systemic sclerosis, dermatomyositis, as complication of subcutaneous or intramuscular injection, etc. Prof. Grases wanted to test the results of topically administered IP$_6$ skin cream on artificially induced dystrophic calcifications in soft tissues. For this experiment the sodium salt of IP$_6$ was chosen over the calcium–magnesium salt due to the higher water solubility of the sodium salt.

As an aside, this study-design also allows the evaluation of the capacity of IP_6 penetration into the organism through the skin

Rats were fed with an IP_6-free or diet with IP_6. Plaque formation was induced by subcutaneous injection of 0.1% $KMnO_4$ solution. From 4 days before plaque induction to the end of the experiment, control rats were treated topically with a standard cream, whereas the experimental rats were treated with the same cream with 2% Na-IP_6. Calcification of plaques was allowed to proceed for 10 days. Topical IP_6 in the moisturizing cream resulted in a statistically significantly reduced plaque size and weight when compared to the control group (1.6 ± 1.1 mg IP_6-treated v 26.7 ± 3.0 mg control). The urinary IP_6 levels of animals treated with the IP_6-enriched cream were considerably and significantly higher than those found in animals treated topically with the cream without IP_6 (16.96 ± 4.32 mg L^{-1} IP_6-treated v 0.06 ± 0.03 mg L^{-1} control) indicating the absorption of IP_6 through skin, validating the usefulness of incorporating IP_6 in skin cream for not just *calcinosis cutis* but also in radiation protection such as in sunscreen, moisturizing cream etc.

The other more common and even more painful
examples of pathological calcifications are abnormal stone formation in the kidney, gall bladder,
and less commonly in the salivary glands (sialolithiasis); I discuss them next:

Kidney Stones (Urolithiasis or Renal Calculi)

Patients often tell that passing a kidney stone is
more painful than delivering their children. From
1% to 5% of the population form renal calculi
(stones), of which 80% to 95% of those are composed of calcium oxalate or calcium phosphate.
Fortunately, many do not experience symptoms, or
pass small sand-like sediments or stones with no
complications. Unfortunately, for those that do
manage to get a stone lodged in the ureter, which
is the tube running to the bladder from the kidney,
they often have a tale of severe pain to tell.

Back in 1958 Dr. Philip Henneman and his associates at Harvard Medical School and Massachusetts
General Hospital in Boston published the clinical
results of 35 men using IP₆ in *The New England
Journal of Medicine*. The patients had normal
blood levels of calcium, but increased levels in

their urine (idiopathic hypercalciuria), which is the main risk factor for kidney stones. The men took 8.8 grams of sodium IP₆ orally in divided doses. The patients' urinary calcium levels returned to normal; 10 of the patients took IP₆ for an extended period (on average 24 months) and only 2 of these 10 developed a kidney stone. **IP₆ normalized the hypercalciuria and significantly lessened kidney stone growth and recurrence.** The treatment of the day was a low calcium diet (avoidance of dairy) and increased fluid intake, which offered limited success. This begs the question: why, when a safe and much more effective treatment was revealed, it was not followed up and investigated further (even with the fame and prestige of Harvard Medical School, Massachusetts General Hospital and worldwide circulation of *The New England Journal of Medicine*!)?

As if 'it is never too late', four decades later, Prof. Grases presented research at the Kyoto Japan *"First International Symposium on Disease Prevention by IP₆ and Other Components of Rice"*. Prof. Grases showed a significant inhibition of calcium oxalate crystallization, which is a key event required in kidney stone formation with IP₆ in an *in vitro* study. In a clinical study with 74 patients (who were calcium oxalate stone formers) he and his colleagues showed that the risk of calcium stone formation was reduced within 2 weeks after being treated with 120 mg of calcium-magnesium IP$_6$ (Lit-Stop™) daily in contrast to the control patients. Note that the dose of 120 mg is much lower than used in the Harvard study performed decades earlier.

About a half-century after Dr Henneman's publication from Harvard University, in April 2004, Dr. Gary C. Curhan and his associates, also at Harvard, published results from the Nurses Health Study II. The women filled out detailed food frequency questionnaires in 1991 and 1995. The 96,245 women had no prior history of kidney stones. The enormous size of this study group is highly significant, as results occurring due to chance are very unlikely. The researchers prospectively examined during an 8 year period the association between dietary factors and the risk of symptomatic kidney stones. There were two main conclusions from the study, both of which were very interesting.

First, "**A higher intake of dietary calcium decreases the risk of kidney stone formation in younger women, but supplemental calcium is not associated with risk**". This finding completely contradicts the strategy of limiting calcium intake as has often been suggested. Secondly, and highly relevant to our discussion was this concluding statement: *"Finally, dietary phytate [IP₆] may be a new, important, and safe addition to our options for stone prevention."*

Kidney stone incidence has been rising since the late 19th century in Europe and North America as well as in Japan since World War II. The rise in kidney stone incidence correlates closely with dietary change towards a more refined diet, which typically offers less IP_6. It is estimated that approximately 5% of American women and 12% of men will have a kidney stone at some time in life with an estimated cost of $2.1 billion annually, not to mention of the pain and suffering.

Hospitalization statistics of South African Blacks provides more convincing evidence as to the value of IP_6 containing foods for the prevention of kidney stones. From 1971 to 1979 Dr. Monte Modlin of the Medical School of Cape Town reported that 1 of every 510 White patients admitted to the school's teaching hospital were for kidney stones. In contrast, only 1 of 44,298 Black admissions was for kidney stones. **That's almost a 90-fold difference!** In Cape Town in 1970, 5.1 million Blacks and 4.5 million Whites lived in the urban areas. For Blacks moving from the rural to urban areas it generally results in a more "city-like" diet. However, the Black-people's diet is still based on daily maize or corn consumption of about 680 grams, especially in the first generation of new city dwellers. As corn may contain up to 6% IP₆, it works out to be *up to* a whopping 40.8 grams of IP₆ daily [please keep in mind that not all of it is absorbed as discussed earlier].

There are four main types of kidney stones: i) the vast majority (approximately 70%) are calcium-containing, either calcium oxalate (CaOx) or a mixture of calcium oxalate + calcium phosphate (CaP); ii) about 15% are the so-called triple stones (aka struvite stones); iii) uric acid stone (5% - 10%) and finally iv) the rare (1%-2%) cysteine stones. The most important determinant is an increased urinary concentration of the stones' constituents to the point that the urine becomes supersaturated. A simple analogy is trying to mix salt or sugar in a glass of water; if the amount of salt is small it dissolves and you do not see it; but if you add too much salt you reach a point when the water is no longer able to dissolve the excess salt and now you can see the salt as insoluble precipitate. You can dissolve the extra salt or sugar by either adding more water (so drink plenty of water!) or adding something to the mixture that will remove the extra salt/sugar. IP$_6$ is one such substance that removes the extra calcium from the urine.

However, the formation of kidney stones involves *both* an alteration in the composition of the urine and damages in the renal tissue such as necrosis, calcification etc. Thus, not all people with high blood calcium or citrate or uric acid level will develop a kidney stone unless their kidneys have some damaged tissue as well. In the very first step a crystal has to form, then it has to grow and then many such growing crystals have to aggregate to each other before it becomes large enough to become a fully-grown stone.

Approximately 1 to 3% of ingested IP$_6$ leaves the body via the urine (the majority of the IP$_6$ is used by the cells and eventually gets broken down and in fact is expired out the lungs as carbon dioxide or CO$_2$; Sakamoto *et al* 1993, Nahapetian & Young 1980). Prof. Grases' experiments point to IP$_6$'s inhibition of crystallization as the mechanism for kidney stone prevention. IP$_6$ exiting out the kidneys is able to bind and remove calcium atoms that make up or are part of kidney stones. Bound together, IP$_6$ and excess calcium are then both eliminated from the body via the urine. A kidney stone contains millions of atoms of calcium. Thus, it is like removing a single grain of sand, after single grain of sand, and so on and so on from a sandbox. Eventually the sandbox will be emptied as will the kidney stone be slowly dissolved.

Additional studies by Saw *et al* (2007) have shown that IP_6 can remove calcium from the artificial urine by about half at 2.2 mM concentration. In addition to decreasing the level of ionized calcium, IP_6 enhances the barrier to heterogeneous nucleation, inhibits its crystallization activity and inhibits *in vitro* stone growth. Thus, IP_6 provides a safe and effective treatment. It is simply a case of having enough IP_6 in the urine to do the job.

If you've had a kidney stone, chances are you'll have another. As such, a preventive strategy is called for. Current therapy often includes an increased water intake, often combined with a diuretic. IP_6+inositol provides a whole new and safe approach. If you are fortunate enough to have never had an episode, this supplement is likely your best insurance aside from eating a simple, healthful diet. This stone preventive aspect of IP_6+inositol as yet another of its multiple benefits.

Sialolithiasis (Salivary Gland Stone)

Sialolithiasis means calcific stone formation in the ducts of the salivary glands, most commonly in the submandibular gland. As expected, these stones result in pain and blockage of the salivary duct with resultant inflammation, causing more pain. Prof. Grases and his team chemically analyzed 21 such stones and the saliva from the patients whose stones they analyzed. Salivary calcium was significantly higher in 18 of the 21 patients. More interestingly, IP_6 concentration in the saliva of these 18 patients was significantly lower than that found in saliva of healthy individuals. This study shows that IP_6 is present in the normal saliva, and thus taking IP_6 supplement could raise salivary IP_6 content and help prevent sialolithiasis. ***"It was concluded that the deficit of crystallization inhibitors such as myo-inositol hexaphosphate (phytate [IP₆]) was also an important etiologic factor implied in the sialolith development (F. Grases** et **al.** 2003).*

Having discussed the presence of IP_6 in saliva and its role in prevention of stone in salivary gland, let us now move to the other more conspicuous and important structure – our teeth.

Erosion of the Teeth

The pH of saliva should ideally be between 6.5 and 5.5. It is generally believed that the pH of 5.5 is the threshold for developing dental caries. Prolonged exposure to <pH 5.5, or frequent cycling from optimal (neutral) pH to below the threshold (pH 5.5) can result in rapid demineralization of the enamel. Lowered salivary pH is often a result of bacterial digestion of various sugars such as sucrose, fructose etc. This causes accumulation of acidic byproducts in the dental plaques. The consumption of citrus fruits and soft-drinks may be a major factor in causing dental erosion which is an irreversible process.

Carbonated soft-drinks have a low pH and contain sugar and other additives thereby putting the enamel at a very high risk of dissolution and/ or erosion. In the pathogenesis of dental erosion, it is the total acid level called titratable acidity, rather than the pH that is considered important (Hara & Zero 2008).

The high ingestion of soft-drinks poses a major public health problem not just in the USA, but globally as it is replacing milk consumption, thus reducing the recommended dietary intake of calcium.

Hara & Zero (2008) thus investigated whether added calcium to the beverages would affect their enamel-erosive action. Ten commercially available beverages, 5 with and 5 without calcium supplementation were tested. They demonstrate a lower level of enamel demineralization with calcium supplemented beverages.

von Fraunhofer & Rogers (2004) examined the relative rate of enamel dissolution in a variety of carbonated soft-drinks. Caries-free human teeth were placed in *Coca Cola, Pepsi Cola, Dr. Pepper, Mountain Dew, Ginger Ale* and *Sprite* for 14 days. The cola beverages (*Coca Cola, Pepsi Cola* and *Dr. Pepper*) showed enamel dissolution (weight loss) of about 3 mg/cm^2 whereas, the non-cola drinks (*Mountain Dew, Ginger Ale* and *Sprite*) showed a 2-5 times greater dissolution! Jain *et al* (2007) also showed that prolonged exposure to soft drinks can lead to significant enamel loss, and that the non-cola drinks are more erosive than cola drinks. Cola and non-cola drinks with sugar were more erosive than their diet counterparts.

As you very well know, soft-drinks are extremely popular not just in the developed countries, but thanks to effective marketing and promotion, in the developing world as well. In the United States alone, the yearly sale has been estimated to be over $65 billion with a 30% annual growth rate! The omnipresent vending machines, now also in the schools, are making the consumption even higher, particularly amongst young adults and children. Most soft-drinks are acidic in pH and their exposure to teeth may result in enamel erosion; no wonder, our children have poor dental health.

How can IP_6 help? Experiments with IP_6 have shown that addition of IP_6+inositol reduced the % titratable acidity (TA) of soft drinks. Subsequent studies have shown that additions of IP_6+inositol to a variety of beverages, including *Fresca* and *Red Bull*, reduce the % TA to close to 0. Further studies were performed on extracted human teeth, either on sections of enamel dissected off the crowns or intact teeth with the root portion of the teeth beneath the enamel/dentin junction coated with protective varnish. These enamel specimens were immersed in the various soft drinks with or without additions of 0.5 and 1.0% by weight of IP_6. The enamel dissolution was determined as the weight loss of the enamel at different time intervals in the untreated and treated beverages Shamsuddin & von Fraunhofer 2007).

As can be seen in the following Figures, addition of IP_6 results in marked protection of the teeth from the erosive effect of soft-drinks. One option to deliver IP_6 is to simply add it to the drinks. IP_6 could also be provided in small paper packages as for salt & pepper found in coffee shops, restaurant tables etc.

And of course, as Prof. Grases has shown, even orally administered IP_6 is protective of the salivary gland stones; IP_6 must be excreted therein to serve its function. But a more direct approach such as addition to the drinks, either at the time of manu-facturing or at the time of consumption may be the ideal way to prevent dental erosion.

Titratable acidity

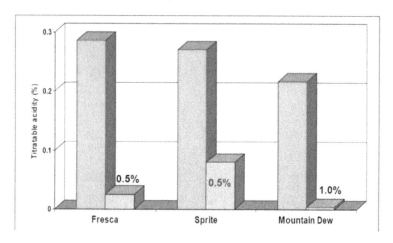

Figure 14-1. The protective effect of IP₆ (0.5% and 1%) as reduction in titratable acidity against *Fresca*, *Sprite* and *Mountain Dew* is shown here.

An additional advantage of IP₆ supplement is the availability of calcium-magnesium IP₆. As Hara & Zero (2008) tell us, even supplemental calcium by itself can reduce the enamel erosion.

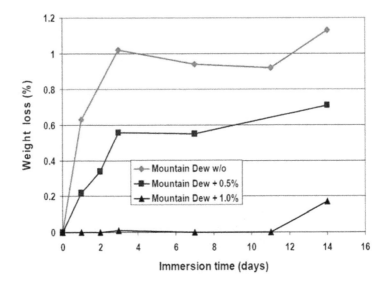

Figure 14-2: Addition of IP₆ results in decreased weight loss (enamel erosion) by *Mountain Dew*; higher concentration of IP₆ confers even better protection.

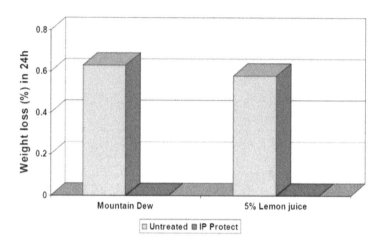

Figure 14-3: IP₆ (red or darker almost non-existent right-hand columns) dramatically prevents the enamel erosion as measured by weight loss from Mountain Dew or 5% lemon juice; left hand columns are control untreated samples.

Thus calcium-magnesium IP₆ provides double protection by providing calcium as well as IP₆. What could be better?!

CHAPTER 15

NEURO-
PSYCHIATRIC
DISORDERS

Alzheimer's Disease (AD)

In 1907 the German psychiatrist and neuropatho-
logist Dr. Alois Alzheimer described a dementia in
the elderly eponymously known as Alzheimer's
disease (AD), the commonest type of dementia in
our seniors today. It is not a new disease by any
means. The ancient Greek and Roman philosoph-
ers had noted increasing dementia along with adv-

ancing age. Pathological hallmark of the disease is loss of nerve cells (neurons) and their communicating junctions with each other (synapses) in the brain resulting in its shrinkage (atrophy); the characteristic lesions are **neurofibrillary tangles** and **amyloid plaques.** The tangles are aggregates of the microtubule-associated protein *tau* which has become hyper-phosphorylated and accumulate within the cells. Although many older individuals develop some plaques and tangles as a consequence of aging, the brains of AD patients have a greater number of them in specific areas. It can be considered as disease of protein misfolding as the amyloid plaques are composed of misfolded β-amyloid protein (Aβ). Aβ is found in extracellular deposits throughout the central nervous system; insofar as to our understanding of how the disease starts, this is where the consensus ends. Neither my intention, nor the purpose of the book is to delve into the controversies of AD pathogenesis; thus, I shall restrict to the information relevant to IP_6 and inositol.

Let's bring Prof. Fèlix Grases for the last time! In January 2010 he put forward a tantalizing hypothesis, based on the observation that the pineal gland hormone melatonin level decreases with advancing age, but more so in AD patients. This somewhat neglected melatonin has multiple important roles aside from being an antioxidant and a neuroprotective agent; even more to the point is that melatonin inhibits the formation $A\beta$. But why does the pineal gland stops secreting this crucial neuroprotectant? That the pineal gland, the source of our melatonin becomes calcified correlating with decreased secretion of melatonin with age is well known. We know that calcification may take place if there is a lack of inhibitors of calcium salt crystallization, of which IP_6 is one. Thus, Prof. Grases and colleagues propose that IP_6 deficiency may be a risk factor for AD.

Interestingly exactly a year later, in January 2011 a paper came out in the *Journal of Alzheimer's Disease* proposing treatment of AD with IP_6. $A\beta$ is believed to interfere with neuronal activity because of its stimulatory effect on the production of **free radicals, resulting in oxidative stress and neuronal cell death.** Dr. Thimmappa Anekonda and colleagues at the Oregon Health & Science University in Portland, and Superfox Therapeutics in New York, thus tested the ability of IP_6 in preventing $A\beta$-induced pathology in both *in vitro* and *in vivo* models of AD. Human neuroblastoma MC65 cells were used for *in vitro* and Tg2576 mouse model for *in vivo* studies. They show that IP_6 protects MC65 cells against the harmful effect of Aβ and caused a modest reduction in the level of Aβ and plaques in the Tg2576 mice treated with IP$_6$.

Needless to state that considering the frustrating lack of any remedies, preventive or therapeutic, and the devastation that AD causes, this is a very encouraging report, one that shows great promise for combating this scourge simply by IP$_6$.

But hold on! Not to be left out, inositol may have something to say here too! Noting that a) inositol is dysregulated in Down's syndrome and AD, b) uptake of *myo*-inositol is increased in the fibroblast cells in Down's, and c) a large amount of Aβ is present in the brain of Down's syndrome patients prior to the deposition of plaques, Prof. JoAnne McLaurin and her colleagues at the University of Toronto, Canada have studied the 4 stereoisomers of inositol to see if inositol will have any effect on AD. They used PC-12[1] cells and primary human neuronal culture to answer their questions. Their results show that inositol interacts with Aβ; the resultant Aβ-inositol complex is non-toxic to both [nerve growth factor-differentiated] PC-12 cells

---

[1] Pheochromocytoma cells from rat adrenal medulla. In response to nerve growth factors these cells stop growing and terminally differentiate, making them a good model to study nerve cells.

and primary human neuronal cultures. The investigators believe that the reduction of toxicity is the result of Aβ-inositol interaction. Since inositol stereoisomers are naturally occurring molecules that readily cross the blood-brain barrier they further believe that inositols may represent a viable treatment for AD.

> "...*inositol treatment for AD patients may help to prevent Aβ-deposition and Aβ-induced toxicity*" (**McLaurin** et al, **2000**).

They further expanded their investigation to TgCRND8 mice, a model for AD with *scyllo*-inositol and confirmed their earlier *in vitro* findings.

Notwithstanding the use of a different isomer of inositol in this study, the exact logic for which is a bit unclear to me, the preceding, also begs for the combination of IP₆+Inositol in prevention and perhaps therapy of AD.

Parkinson's Disease (PD)

Parkinson's disease (PD) is another debilitating neurological disease that affects an estimated 1%

of the population of 50 years of age in USA. Characteristic microscopic finding is selective degeneration of dopaminergic cells in special area of the brain called *substantia nigra* and *locus ceruleus*. Usual residents of these areas are cells with dark pigment (hence the name *substantia nigra*) who become degenerated, dead and replaced by gliosis, a special form of brain fibrosis with resultant irreversible motor dysfunction. Since the basic pathology is loss of dopamine producing cells, the treatment option is dopamine replacement therapy, which only gives symptomatic relief as the cells are irreversibly lost.

How and why do these cells undergo degeneration and die? If we could find the answer to these how and why then we could certainly prevent this disease. It turns out that oxidative damage may be a causative factor in the pathogenesis of PD. By now we know that IP₆ and inositol are great antioxidants who have multiple health benefits. Experimentally, 1-methyl-4-phenyl 1,2,3,6-tetra-hydropyridine (MPTP) produces a Parkinson's syndrome after its conversion to a dopamine-selective neurotoxin 1-methyl-4-phenylpyridini-um ion (MPP$^+$) through the formation of •OH. Thus, Dr. Toshio Obata of Oita Medical University in Japan set out to investigate if IP₆ would have any potential bene-

fit in PD in an *in vivo* rat model. Their study showed that IP_6 significantly suppressed iron-enhanced
MPP^+-induced •OH formation (Obata 2003).

Using an *in vitro* model system, Dr. Manju Reddy
and her colleagues at the Iowa State University in
Ames, USA also have used rat brain cells that
produce dopamine, induced their damage and cell
death (apoptosis) and tested with IP_6. Compared to
the control non-IP_6 treated cells, treatment of these
cells with IP_6 resulted in a 22% decrease in cell
death, data being statistically significant at $p<0.05$.
Other measurements of cell damage and apoptosis
parameters showed even higher level of protection
encouraging the scientists to conclude:

> "...*our results demonstrate a significant
> neuroprotective effect of phytate [IP₆] in a
> cell culture model.*" (Xu *et al Toxicology*
> 2008).

The authors further report in the journal *Parkinson's Disease* published online on 7 February
2011, that IP_6 protects against 6-hydroxy-dopa-
mine-induced cell apoptosis in both normal and
iron-excess conditions in immortalized rat mesen-
cephalic dopaminergic neuronal cell line (1RB3-

AN27 also known as N27), "and IP6 may offer neuroprotection in PD."

Psychiatric Disorders

Brain has one of the highest levels of IP_6, and it has been considered to play a role in neuronal signaling. In the late 1980's and early 1990's IP_6 was found to stimulate Ca^{2+} uptake in cultured cerebellar neurons and anterior pituitary cells. Moreover, the low concentration of IP_6 increases both intracellular free Ca^{2+} and prolactin secretion in perifused pituitary cells. Subsequently, IP_6–binding sites, the IP_6 receptor was isolated. Radiolabelled IP_6 ($[^3H]$-IP_6) bound to specific and saturable recognition sites in membranes prepared from cerebral hemispheres, anterior pituitaries and cultured cerebellar neurons in all subcellular fractions including the mitochondria. On the other hand, the level of *myo*-inositol in brain cells is reduced in a variety of neuropsychiatric conditions. The level of inositol in cerebrospinal fluid (that bathes the brain and the spinal cord) has been found to be reduced in patients with depression. And experimentally, injection of inositol inside the ventricular cavity in the brain reverses seizures in animals.

Furthermore, large doses of inositol injected inside the body cavity raises the inositol level in the cerebrospinal fluid and can also reverse seizures in experimental animals. Clinically, inositol level is decreased in the cerebrospinal fluid of patients with depression.

"Demonstration that inositol enters the brain after peripheral administration provides a basis for pharmacological intervention in psychiatric disorders" conclude the authors (Agam **et al** *1994).*

Two clinical trials have shown that large amounts of inositol can improve mental depression. A double-blind controlled clinical trial was performed at the Ben Gurion University of the Negev by the Israeli Ministry of Health on clinically depressed patients. When 28 depressed patients were given 12 grams of inositol a day, a statistically significant overall benefit was found for inositol treatment when compared to the placebo group. This improvement was detected as early as week 4 on the Hamilton Depression scale, the standard measure to assess the effectiveness of an antidepressant substance (Levine, 1977).

The conventional treatments for patients with anxiety disorders in the United States include antidepressants which are not without their own side-effects such as sleep disturbances, sexual dysfunction, gastrointestinal problems, weight gain etc. In that regard, natural remedies may be more appealing and inositol offers itself to that service!

Panic disorder

The following two studies also from Israel should be convincing enough:

Benjamin *et al* (1995) examined the effectiveness of inositol versus placebo in panic disorder in a double-blind crossover trial involving 21 patients. The patients were assigned to either 12g/day of inositol or placebo for 4 weeks each. All of the patients then crossed over to the alternate treatment arm for additional 4 weeks. The baseline number of panic attacks per week for all subjects was 9.7±15, which decreased to 3.7±4 in subjects taking inositol (significant at P=.04) as opposed to 6.3±9 in the placebo arm. The mean scores of severity of panic attacks also decreased significantly from 72±140 at baseline for all subjects to

31 ± 50 during the placebo arm and to 11 ± 11 during inositol treatment; the difference being quite significant at $P=0.007$).

In another study by the same group, 20 patients with panic disorder with or without agoraphobia (extreme fear of open space) were given either inositol (up to 18/day) or fluvoxamine (up to 150 mg/day) for 4 weeks in a double-blind, controlled, random-order crossover study (Palatnik *et al* 2001). Compared to the conventional drug fluvoxamine that decreased weekly panic attacks from 5.8 ± 4 at baseline to 3.4 ± 4 at endpoint, the frequency of panic attacks in the patients in inositol group decreased from 7.2 ± 4 to 3.1 ± 3. Statistical analysis showed that the inositol was marginally more effective than fluvoxamine from baseline to endpoint for treating the number of panic attacks ($P=.049$). The two treatments were considered equally effective at reducing Hamilton Anxiety scores, agoraphobia scores, and Clinical Global Impression of Severity (CGI-S) scores. Not unexpectedly, side effects were minimal with inositol treatment, as opposed to frequent nausea and tiredness associated fluvoxamine. 'All things considered', inositol was more effective than fluvoxamine in reducing the number of panic attacks with less adverse effects (Palatnik *et al* 2001).

Obsessive-Compulsive Disorder (OCD)

The effectiveness of inositol in OCD was studied in 13 patients in a double-blind controlled cross-over trial of 18g/day of inositol or placebo for 6 weeks each. The patients had significantly lower scores on the Y-BOCS[2] when taking inositol than when taking placebo (*P*=.009) (Fux *et al* 1996).

Carey *et al* (2004) in Cape Town, South Africa studied the effect of inositol treatment on brain function in OCD through single-photon emission computed tomography. Fourteen subjects underwent single-photon emission computed tomography before and after receiving inositol for 12 weeks. Following treatment with inositol, there was deactivation in OCD responders relative to non-responders in several areas of the brain with significant reductions in Y-BOCS and CGI-S[3] scores. These results not only show the efficacy of inositol in OCD, but also suggest that inositol may exert its clinical effects through alternate neuronal circuitry to the selective serotonin reuptake inhibitors (SSRIs) – the anti-depressants.

---

[2] Yale-Brown obsessive compulsive scale tests the severity of OCD
[3] Clinical global impression scale commonly used measures of symptom severity, treatment-response and the efficacy of treatments in studies of patients with mental disorders.

EPILOGUE

"If this IP_6+inositol is as good as it appears to be, then why is this not being widely used or sold by the drug companies?!" That's a question I am often asked, mostly with sarcasm, but sometimes as innocent curiosity. Whichever is your motive, please allow me to shed some light.

In the United States and most of the developed countries, drugs for the treatment of cancer or other diseases have to be extensively tested in the laboratory and then in humans as clinical trials and found to have met the criteria for acceptance by the regulatory agencies (e.g. Food and Drug Administration – FDA in USA). Compared to the preclinical laboratory testing, the clinical trials are enormously expensive, tens of millions of dollars in the USA. Drug companies with deep pocket who see a good return of their investment would sponsor such trials with the aim of making good profit, naturally. So, natural products are out of the question; while one would not hesitate to come up with $10 for a pill for erectile dysfunction, paying even $1 for a capsule of IP$_6$+Inositol would be a tough sell. So why should the drug companies be interested? Then comes the U.S. National Cancer Institute (NCI) who occasionally sponsors promising drugs for cancer treatment. Unfortunately, the NCI had decided some time ago that IP$_6$ does not work in their system using concentrations 100- to 10,000-fold less (!) than what we and others throughout the world have been using. NCI's handling of this subject was adequately covered in the book *"Too Good to be True?!"* by Drs. Kim Vanderlinden and Ivana Vucenik. Suffice it to say that NCI's final 'blow' was their position that "anti-cancer drugs must be administered intravenously and not orally" ...since IP$_6$ is given orally, NCI had no interest in it. Hence there was no sponsoring of clinical trial of IP$_6$. But, I would be remiss if I did not mention that NCI *has* been funding research on IP$_6$ and inositol, albeit limited and for basic research; some of the studies described (e.g. Professors Agarwal, Pretlow etc.) were NCI sponsored.

I agree with many who think that Mother Nature or God, whatever one chooses to believe in, has provided us with all that we need to solve our problems. Consider all the major categories of drugs: aspirin, antibiotics, drugs for heart disease (digi-

talis), for malaria (quinine) etc. that has been identified in nature. So when I look at IP_6 and inositol,
I wonder why are they everywhere? They are in
the soil from where they go through the roots and
stems of plants to the cereals and legumes; cereals
(rice, corn, wheat, soybean etc.) constitute the sta-
ple diet of much of the population in our planet.
And then they are in all of the mammalian cells
that have been tested so far. So why are they ubi-
quitous or omnipresent?

Clearly, deficiency of IP_6 is associated with increased risk of various diseases and adequate supplementation reverses those conditions. These characteristics argue strongly for its inclusion as a vitamin.

About half-a-century ago, Morton and Raison first
suggested a link between IP_6 and ATP regenera-
tion and its importance in seed development and
germination. As usual, there was considerable ske-
pticism to such 'outlandish' ideas. It was not till
1978 that the hypothesis appeared more plausible:
an IP_6 – ADP phosphotransferase described by
Biswas *et al* could use IP_6 as a phosphate donor for
the conversion of ADP to ATP by transferring a
phosphate group from 2 position of IP_6 to ADP in
developing mung bean *Phaseolus aureus* seeds.

Additional support came from Phillippy *et al* who isolated an inositol 1,3,4,5,6-pentakisphosphate 2-kinase which is involved in both formation of IP$_6$ in maturing seeds and catalyze the conversion of ATP from ADP in germinating seeds, in this case the soybean. It should not be an 'outlandish' idea to think that in mammalian cells too, IP$_6$ may be crucial in providing the phosphates so necessary in the conversion of ADP $\rightarrow$ ATP, the fundamental 'transaction of currency' that drives the cells and the organism to action; almost everything we or our cells do need energy and conversion of ADP $\rightarrow$ ATP and the reverse gives us the power to do what we want or need. A good analogy would be IP$_6$ as the money or credit/debit card that pays for your gasoline (ADP $\rightarrow$ ATP) to allow you to drive!

In this age of easy access to information one can readily get the latest research results *via* the Internet, let alone the news media that more often than not, overhype the news especially when it comes to health matters. This may cause information-overload. It has become a tendency for many to take isolated research data on a single step in the biochemical process of the cell (there are numerous steps and processes) and then apply it for their dietary habits or treatment choices, completely ignoring the fact that our body is infinitely more complex, with interactions between various 'systems' as well as being provided with checks & balances and adaptations etc. I sincerely hope that you will not lose this perspective having read this book. The book is intended to provide you with authentic scientific information; hopefully it will help you make informed decision about your own health and wellbeing.

Too good to be true?! If you have lingering doubts, then perhaps you might want to check it out yourself. There are several entities that are marketing the products; unfortunately, the purity, potency and hence the quality of these varies strikingly. To begin with there are some who are marketing only IP₆. As you have seen in the breast and colon cancer studies, the ***combination of IP₆ and inositol in proper proportion*** yields the best results both for cancer prevention as well for boosting the NK cell activity. Thus, marketing something for human health that is not optimal is irresponsible at best. Then there is the issue of purity and potency. The raw material calcium-magnesium IP₆ comes in a range of 50-97% purity. Naturally, the purer the material, the more potent and the more expensive it is. To lure uninformed and thrifty consumers, many marketers are selling the IP₆ that are abo-

ut 50% pure! Currently, Seymour Biotech
(www.SeymourBiotech.com) is the manufacturer
of the highest quality of IP$_6$ products. Besides their
IP6+Inositol, and *IP6 Health*, products with lab-
els bearing either of the following logos have my
endorsement:

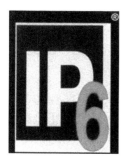
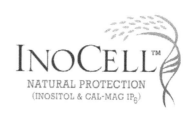

For updated research information, directly pertine-
nt to health benefits, you may wish to periodically
visit www.ip-6.net.

How much to take? Unbelievable as it may seem,
over a quarter of a century since the first demonstration of its anticancer function a phase I clinical
trial for dose-determination is yet to be performed!
Hence, the following guideline has been extrapo-
lated from experimental data. I believe that a total
of about 2gm IP$_6$ + Inositol (4 capsules) in two divided doses is a reasonable amount for otherwise
healthy individuals; that's what I have been taking

every day since 1998. I am happy to share with you that during this period I have not had a single episode of flu [and have not been taking the 'flu-shot' either], or even common cold. Don't forget, prevention is just as important if not more than treatment. About the latter, therapeutic doses would be approximately 4-6 times more. An intermediate dose may be appropriate for disease-free high-risk individuals.

Good Health!

2 gm /2 = 1g for 2x a day

2 gm total

BIBLIOGRAPHY

Abelson, P. H.: A potential phosphate crisis. *Science* 283: 2015-2016. 1999.

Agam, G., Shapiro, Y., Bersudsky, Y., Kofman, O, Bell-marker, R. H.: High-dose peripheral inositol raises brain inositol levels and reverses behavioral effects of inositol depletion by lithium. *Pharmacology, Biochemistry & Behavior*. 49: 341-343, 1994.

Agarwal, C., Dhanalakshmi, S., Singh, R. P., and Agarwal, R.: Inositol hexaphosphate inhibits growth and induces G1 arrest and apoptotic death of androgen-dependent human prostate carcinoma LNCaP cells. *Neoplasia* 6:646-659. 2004.

Agarwal, C., Dhanalakshmi, S., Singh, R. P., and Agarwal, R.: Inositol hexaphosphate inhibits constitutive activation of NF- kappa B in androgen-independent human prostate carcinoma DU145 cells. *Anticancer Research* 23:3855-3861, 2003.

Aljandali, A., Pollack, H., Yeldandi, A, Weitzman S. A., Kamp, D.W.: Asbestos causes apoptosis in alveolar epithelial cells: role of iron-induced free radicals. *J Lab Clin Med* 137: 330-339, 2001.

Amaral, E. G., Fagundes, D. J., Marks, G., and Inouye, C.
M.: Study of superoxide dismutase's expression in
the colon produced by azoxymethane and inositol
hexaphosfate's paper, in mice. *Acta Cir Bras* 21
Supplement 4: 27-31, 2006.

Anekonda, T.S., Wadsworth, T.L., Sabin, R., Frahler, K.,
Harris, C., Petriko, B, Ralle, M., Woltjer, R., Quinn,
J.F. Phytic acid as a potential treatment for
Alzheimer's pathology: evidence from animal and
in vitro models. *J of Alzheimer's Disease* 23: 21-35,
2011.

Arnold, J. T., Wilkinson, B. P., Sharma, S., and Steele, V.
E.: Evaluation of chemopreventive agents in
different mechanistic classes using a rat tracheal
epithelial cell culture transformation assay. *Cancer Research* 55:537-543, 1995.

Babich, H., Borenfreund, E., and Stern, A.: Comparative
cytotoxicities of selected minor dietary non-nutri-
ents with chemopreventive properties. *Cancer
Letters* 73:127-133, 1993 .

Bacić, I., Drzijanić, N., Karlo, R., Skifić, I., Jagić, S.:
Efficacy of IP6 + Inositol in the treatment of
breast cancer patients receiving chemotherapy:
prospective, randomized, pilot clinical study.
*Journal of Experimental and Clinical Cancer
Research* 29: 12, 2010.

Baghurst, P. A., and Rohan, T. E.: High-fiber diets and reduced risk of breast cancer. *International Journal of Cancer* 56:173-176, 1994.

Baten, A., Ullah, A., Tomazic, V. J., and Shamsuddin, A. M.: Inositol phosphate induced enhancement of natural killer cell activity correlates with tumor suppression. *Carcinogenesis* 10: 1595-1598, 1989.

Benjamin, J., Agam, G., Levine, J., Bersudsky, Y., Kofman, O., and Belmaker, R. H.: Inositol treatment in psychiatry. *Psychopharmacol Bull.* 31:167-75. 1995.

Benjamin, J., Levine, J., Fux, M., Aviv, A., Levy, D., and Belmarker, R.H. Double-blind, placebo-controlled, cross-over trial of inositol treatment for panic disorder. *Am J Psychiatry* 152:1084-1086, 1995.

Berridge, M. J., and Irvine, R. F.: Inositol phosphates and cell signalling. *Nature* 341:197-205, 1989.

Bingham, S. A., Day, N. E., Luben, R., *et al.*; European Prospective Investigation into Cancer and Nutrition: Dietary fibre in food and protection against colorectal cancer in the European Prospective Investigation into Cancer and Nutrition (EPIC): an observational study. [see comment] [Erratum *Lancet* 2003 Sep 20;362(9388):1000]. *Lancet* 361:1496-1501. 2003.

Biswas, S., Maity, I. B., Chakrabarti, S., and Biswas, B. B.:
Purification and characterization of myo-inositol
hexaphosphate-adenosine diphosphate phosphotransferase from *Phaseolus aureus. Arch Biochem
Biophys*. 185: 557-566. 1978.

Bohn, L., Josefsen, L., Meyer, A. S., and Rasmussen, S. K.:
Quantitative analysis of phytate globoids isolated
from wheat bran and characterization of their
sequential dephosphorylation by wheat phytase.
Journal of Agricultural & Food Chemistry
55:7547-7552, 2007.

Bohn, L., Meyer, A. S., and Rasmussen, S. K.: Phytate:
impact on environment and human nutrition. A
challenge for molecular breeding. *Journal of Zhe-
jiang University. Science. B* 9:165-191, 2008.

Bozsik, A., Kökény, S., and Olah, E.: Molecular
mechanisms for the antitumor activity of inositol
hexakis-phosphate (IP6). *Cancer Genomics &
Proteomics* 4: 43-51, 2007.

Burkitt, D. P.: Epidemiology of cancer of the colon and
rectum. *Cancer* 28:3-13, 1971.

Campbell, S., Fisher, R.J., Towler, E.M., Fox, S., Issaq,
H.J., Wolfe, T., Phillips, L.R., and Rein, A.:
Modulation of HIV-like particle assembly *in vitro*
by inositol phosphates. *Proc Natl Acad Sci USA* 98:
10875-10879, 2001

Carey, P. D., Warwick J., Harvey, B. H., Stein, D. J., and Seedat, S.: Single photon emission computed tomography (SPECT) of anxiety disorders before and after treatment with citalopram. *BMC Psychiatry* 4:30. 2004.

Carroll, J. S., Lynch, D. K., Swarbrick, A., Renoir, J. M., Sarcevic, B., Daly, R. J., Musgrove, E. A., and Sutherland, R. L.: p27(Kip1) induces quiescence and growth factor insensitivity in tamoxifen-treated breast cancer cells. *Cancer Research* 63:4322-4326, 2003.

Cebrian, D., Tapia, A., Real, A., Morcillo, M. A.: Inositol hexaphosphate: a potential chelating agent for uranium. *Radiation Prot. Dosimetry* 127: 477-479. 2007.

Cecconi, O., Nelson, R. M., Roberts, W. G., Hanasaki, K., Mannori, G., Schultz, C., Ulich, T. R., Aruffo, A., and Bevilacqua, M. P.: Inositol polyanions. Non-carbohydrate inhibitors of L- and P-selectin that block inflammation. *J Biol Chem* 269: 15060-15066, 1994.

Chagpar, A., Evelegh, M., Fritsche, H., Krishnamurthy, S., Hunt, K. K., and Kuerer, H. M.: Prospective evaluation of a novel approach for the use of a quantitative galactose oxidase-Schiff reaction in ductal fluid samples from women with breast carcinoma. *Cancer* 100:2549-2554, 2004.

Challa, A., Rao, D. R., and Reddy, B. S.: Interactive suppression of aberrant crypt foci induced by azoxymethane in rat colon by phytic acid and green tea. *Carcinogenesis* 18:2023-2026, 1997.

Chatenoud, L., Tavani, A., La Vecchia, C., Jacobs, D. R. Jr, Negri, E., Levi, F., and Franceschi, S.: Whole grain food intake and cancer risk. *International Journal of Cancer* 77:24-28, 1998

Chekeni, F. B., Elliott, M. R., Sandilos, J. K., Walk, S. F., Kinchen, J. M., Lazarowski, E. R., Armstrong, A. J., Penuela S, Laird D. W., Salvesen G. S., Isakson B. E., Bayliss, D. A., and Ravichandran K. S.: Pannexin 1 channels mediate 'find-me' signal release and membrane permeability during apoptosis. *Nature*. 467(7317):863-7, 2010.

Cheung, J. C., Salerno, B., and Hanakahi, L. A.: Evidence for an inositol hexakisphosphate-dependent role for Ku in mammalian nonhomologous end joining that is independent of its role in the DNA-dependent protein kinase. *Nucleic Acids Research* 36: 5713-5726, 2008.

Cholewa, K., Parfiniewicz, B., Bednarek, I., Swiatkowska, L., Jezienicka, E., Kierot, J., and Węglarz, L.: The influence of phytic acid on TNF-alpha and its receptors genes' expression in colon cancer Caco-2 cells. *Acta Poloniae Pharmaceutica* 65:75-79, 2008.

Conklin, K. A.: Dietary antioxidants during cancer chemo-
    therapy: impact on chemotherapeutic effectiveness
    and development of side effects. *Nutr Cancer*: 1-
    18, 2000.

Coppolino, C. A. Hexa-citrated phytate and process of
    preparation thereof. US Patent No 7,009,067. 2006

Coppolino C. A. and Shamsuddin A. M.: Phytic citrate
    compounds and process for preparing the same. US
    Patent # 7,517,868. 2009.

Coppolino C. A. and Shamsuddin A. M.: Phytic citrate
    compounds and process for preparing the same. US
    Patent # 7,989,435. 2011.

Cox, G., and Miller, J.D.: Evaluation of the association of
    galactose oxidase-Schiff's reactivity in sputum
    with lung cancer. Presented at the *American Thora-
    cic Society Annual Meeting*, Orlando, Florida,
    U.S.A. May 24, 2004.

Curhan, .G. C., Willett, W. C., Knight, E. L., and Stampfer,
    M.J.: Dietary factors and the risk of kidney stones
    in younger women. Nurse's Health Study II.
    Archives of Internal Medicine 164: 885-891, 2004.

Datta, S. A., Zhao, Z., Clark, P. K., Tarasov, S., Alexan-
    dratos, J. N., Campbell, S. J., Kvaratskhelia, M.,
    Lebowitz, J., Rein, A.: Interactions between HIV-1
    Gag molecules in solution: an inositol phosphate-
    mediated switch. *J Mol Biol* 365: 799-811, 2007.

deGraffenried, L. A., Chandrasekar, B., Friedrichs, W. E., Donzis, E., Silva, J., Hidalgo, M., Freeman, J. W., and Weiss, G. R.: NF-kappa B inhibition markedly enhances sensitivity of resistant breast cancer tumor cells to tamoxifen. *Annals of Oncology* 15: 885-890. 2004.

deGraffenried, L. A., Friedrichs, W. E., Russell, D. H., Donzis, E. J., Middleton, A. K., Silva, J. M., Roth, R. A., and Hidalgo, M.: Inhibition of mTOR activity restores tamoxifen response in breast cancer cells with aberrant Akt Activity. *Clinical Cancer Research* 10:8059-8067, 2004.

Deliliers, G. L., Servida, F., Fracchiolla, N. S., Ricci, C., Borsotti, C., Colombo, G., and Soligo, D.: Effect of inositol hexaphosphate (IP₆) on human normal and leukaemic haematopoietic cells. *British Journal of Haematology* 117:577-587, 2002.

De Rossa, S., Cirillo, P., Paglia, A., *et al.*: Reactive oxygen species and antioxidants in the pathophysiology of cardio-vascular disease: does the actual knowledge justify a clinical approach? *Curr Vasc Pharmacol.* 8: 259-275, 2010

Diallo, J. S., Betton, B., Parent, N., et al.: Enhanced killing of androgen-independent prostate cancer cells using inositol hexakisphosphate in combination with proteasome inhibitors. *British Journal of Cancer* 99:1613-1622, 2008.

Dilworth, L. L., Omoruyi F. O., Simon, *et al.*: The effect of phytic acid on levels of blood glucose and some enzymes of carbohydrate and lipid metabolism. *West Indian Med J.* 54: 102-106, 2005.

Doll, R.: The geographical distribution of cancer. *British Journal of Cancer* 23:1-8, 1969.

Donovan, J. C., Milic, A., and Slingerland, J. M.: Constitutive MEK/MAPK activation leads to p27(Kip1) deregulation and antiestrogen resistance in human breast cancer cells. *Journal of Biological Chemistry* 276:40888-40895, 2001.

Doria, G. L., Calucci L, Pinzino C, Pilu R, Cassani E, and Nielsen E. Phytic acid prevents oxidative stress in seeds: evidence from a maize (*Zea mays L.*) low phytic acid mutant. *J Exp Bot.* 60: 967- 978, 2009.

Dorsey, M., H. Benghuzzi, M. Tucci, and Z. Cason.. Growth and cell viability of estradiol and IP-6 treated Hep-2 laryngeal carcinoma cells. *Biomedical Sciences Instrumentation* 41:205-210, 2005

Druzijanic N, J. J., Perko Z, and Kraljevic D. IP-6 & Inositol: adjuvant to chemotherapy of colon cancer. A pilot clinical trial. *Rev Oncología* 4: (Suppl 1), 171, 2002.

Druzijanic N, J. J., Perko Z, and Kraljevic D. IP6 + Inositol as adjuvant to chemotherapy of colon cancer: Our clinical experience. *Anticancer Research* 24, 3474, 2004.

Duncan, A. M.: The role of nutrition in the prevention of breast cancer. *AACN Clinical Issues* 15:119-135, 2004.

Efanov, A. M., Zaitsev, S. V., and Berggren, P. O.: Inositol hexakisphosphate stimulates non-Ca2+-mediated and primes Ca2+-mediated exocytosis of insulin by activation of protein kinase C. *Proc National Acad. Sci USA* 94:4435-4439, 1997.

Eggleton, P.: Effect of IP₆ on human neutrophil cytokine production and cell morphology. *Anticancer Research* 19:3711-3715, 1999.

Eiseman, J., Lan, J., Guo, J., Joseph, E, and Vucenik, I.: Pharmacokinetics and tissue distribution of inositol hexaphosphate in C.B17 SCID mice bearing human breast cancer xenografts. *Metabolism* April 11, 2011 (Epub ahead of print).

Elsayed, A., Chakravarthy, A., and Shamsuddin, A.: Inositol hexaphosphate from corn decreased the frequency of colorectal cancer in azoxymethane-treated rats. *Laboratory Investigation* 56: 21A, 1987.

Elsayed, A.M., and Shamsuddin, A.M: Detection of altered glycoconjugate in preneoplastic and neoplastic human large intestinal epithelium by galactose oxidase-Schiff sequence. *Laboratory Investigation* 56: 22A, 1987.

Elsayed, A., and Shamsuddin, A.: A strip test for detection of colorectal cancer. *Laboratory Investigation* 56: 22A, 1987.

Elsayed, A., Ullah, A., and Shamsuddin, A.: Post- initiation dietary supplementation with corn derived inositol hexaphosphate (IP₆) inhibits large intestinal carcinogenesis in F-344 rats. *Federation Proceedings* 46: 585, 1987.

El-Sherbiny, Y. M., Cox, M. C., Ismail, Z. A., Shamsuddin, A. M., and Vucenik, I.: G₀/G₁ arrest and S phase inhibition of human cancer cell lines by inositol hexaphosphate (IP₆). *Anticancer Research* 21:2393-2403, 2001.

Estensen, R. D., and Wattenberg, L. W.: Studies of chemopreventive effects of myo-inositol on benzo[a]pyrene-induced neoplasia of the lung and forestomach of female A/J mice. *Carcinogenesis* 14:1975-1977, 1993.

Ferguson, L. R., and Harris, P. J.: Protection against cancer by wheat bran: role of dietary fibre and phytochemicals. *European Journal of Cancer Prevention* 8:17-25, 1999.

Ferry, S., Matsuda, M., Yoshida, H., and Hirata, M.: Inositol hexakisphosphate blocks tumor cell growth by activating apoptotic machinery as well as by inhibiting the Akt/NFkappaB-mediated cell survival pathway. [Erratum: *Carcinogenesis* 24:149, 2003]. *Carcinogenesis* 23: 2031-2041, 2002.

Fox, C. H., and Eberl, M.: Phytic acid (IP6), novel broad spectrum anti-neoplastic agent: a systematic review. *Complementary Therapies in Medicine* 10: 229-234, 2002.

Fux, M., Levine, J., Aviv, A., Belmaker, R.H. Inositol treatment of obsessive–compulsive disorder. *Am J Psychiatry* 153:1219–1221, 1996.

Fux, M., Benjamin, J., Belmaker, R. H.: Inositol versus placebo augmentation of serotonin reuptake inhibitors in the treatment of obsessive–compulsive disorder: a double-blind cross-over study. *Int J Neuropsychopharmacol*; 2:193–195, 1999.

Gee, J. M., Robertson, J. F., Ellis, I. O., and Nicholson, R. I.: Phosphorylation of ERK1/2 mitogen-activated protein kinase is associated with poor response to anti-hormonal therapy and decreased patient survival in clinical breast cancer. *International Journal of Cancer* 95:247-254, 2001.

Graf, E., and Eaton, J. W.: Dietary suppression of colonic cancer. Fiber or phytate? *Cancer* 56:717-718, 1985.

Graf, E., and Eaton, J. W. Antioxidant functions of phytic acid. *Free Radical Biology & Medicine* 8:61-69, 1990.

Grases, F., Simonet, B. M., Vucenik, I., Prieto, R. M., Costa-Bauza, A., March, J. M., and Shamsuddin, A. M.: Absorption and excretion of orally administered inositol hexaphosphate (IP₆ or phytate) in humans. *Biofactors* 15:53-61, 2001.

Grases, F., Simonet, B. M., Vucenik, I., Perelló, J., Prieto, R.M., Shamsuddin, A.M. Effects of exogenous inositol hexakisphosphate (InsP₆) on the levels of InsP₆ and of inositol trisphosphate (InsP₃) in malignant cells, tissues and biological fluids. *Life Sciences* 71:1535-1546, 2002.

Grases, F., Santiago, C., Simonet, B. M., and Costa-Bauzá, A.: Sialolithiasis: mechanism of calculi formation and etiologic factors. *Clinica Chimica Acta – An International Journal of Clinical Chemistry*. 334: 131-136, 2003.

Grases, F., Perelló, J, Isern, B., and Prieto, R. M.: Study of *myo*-inositol hexaphosphate based cream to prevent dystrophic calcinosis cutis. *British Journal of Dermatology* 152:1022-1025, 2005.

Grases, F., Sanchis, P., Perelló, J., Isern, B., Prieto, R. M., Fernández-Palomeque, C., and Torres, J. J.: Effect of crystallization inhibitors on vascular calcifications induced by vitamin D: a pilot study in Sprague-Dawley rats. *Circ J* 71:1152-1156, 2007.

Grases, F., Sanchis, P., Perelló, J., *et al.*: Phytate reduces age-related cardiovascular calcification. *Frontiers in Bioscience* 13: 7115-7122, 2008.

Grases, F., Costa-Bauzà, A., Prieto, R. M.: A potential role for crystallization inhibitors in treatment of Alzheimer's disease. *Medical Hypotheses* 74: 118-119, 2010.

Greiner, R., Farouk, A. E., Carlsson, N. G., and Konietzny, U.: Myo-inositol phosphate isomers generated by the action of a phytase from a Malaysian wastewater bacterium. *The Protein Journal* 26:577-584, 2007.

Gupta, K. P., Singh, J., and Bharathi, R.: Suppression of DMBA-induced mouse skin tumor development by inositol hexaphosphate and its mode of action. *Nutrition & Cancer* 46:66-72, 2003.

Gustafson, A. M., Soldi, R., Anderlind, C., Scholand, M. B., Qian, J., Zhang, X., Cooper, K., Walker, D., McWilliams, A., Liu, G., Szabo, E., Brody, J., Massion, P. P., Lenburg, M. E., Lam, S., Bild, A. H., and Spira, A.: Airway PI3K pathway activation is an early and reversible event in lung cancer development. *Science Translational Medicine* 2(26): 26ra25, 7 April 2010.

Hanakahi, L., Bartlet-Jones, A., M., Chappell, C., Pappin, D., and West, S. C.: Binding of inositol phosphate to DNA-PK and stimulation of double-strand break repair. *Cell* 102:721-729, 2000.

Hara, A. T., and Zero, D. T.: Analysis of the erosive potential of calcium-containing acidic beverages. *Euro J Oral Sci.* 116: 60-65, 2008

Harland, B. F., and D. Oberleas. Phytate in foods. *World Review of Nutrition & Dietetics* 52:235-259, 1987.

Hartig, T. Über das Klebermehl. *Bot Z* 13: 881-882, 1855.

Hartig, T. Weitere Mitteilungen, das Kleibermehl (Aleuron) betreffend. *Bot Z* 14: 257-269, 1856.

Hawkes C. A., Deng, L. H., Shaw, J. E., Nitz, M., McLaurin, J. Small molecule beta-amyloid inhibitors that stabilize protofibrillar structures *in vitro* improve cognition and pathology in a mouse model of Alzheimer's disease. *Eur J Neurosci.* 31(2):203-213, 2010.

Hirose, M., Ozaki, K., Takaba, K. Fukushima, S., Shirai, T., and Ito, N.: Modifying effects of the naturally occurring antioxidants γ-oryzanol, phytic acid, tannic acid and n-tritriacontane-16, 18-dione in a rat wide-spectrum organ carcinogenesis model. *Carcinogenesis* 12:1917-1921, 1991.

Hodge, C. A., Tran, E. J., Noble, K. N., Alcázar- Román, A. R., Ben-Yishay, R., Scarcelli, J.J., Folkmann, A. W., Shav-Tal, Y., Wente, . S. R., and Cole, C. N.: The Dbp5 cycle at the nuclear pore complex during mRNA export I: dbp5 mutants with defects in RNA binding and ATP hydrolysis define key steps for Nup159 and Gle1. *Genes & Development* 25: 1052-1064, 2011.

Hoeijmakers, J. H. J.: DNA damage, ageing and cancer. *New England Journal of Medicine* 361:1475-1485, 2009.

Howell, A.: The endocrine prevention of breast cancer. *Best Practice & Research Clinical Endocrinology & Metabolism* 22:615-623, 2008.

Huang, C., Ma, W. Y., Hecht, S. S., and Dong, Z.: Inositol hexaphosphate inhibits cell transformation and activator protein 1 activation by targeting phosphatidylinositol-3' kinase. [Erratum appears in *Cancer Research* 1997 Nov 15; 57(22):5198]. *Cancer Research* 57:2873-2878, 1997.

Huisamen, B., and Lochner, A.: Inositol polyphosphates and their binding proteins-a short review. *Molecular & Cellular Biochemistry* 157:229-232, 1996.

Ishikawa, T., Nakatsuru, Y., Zarkovic, M., and Shamsuddin, A. M.: Inhibition of skin cancer by IP₆ *in vivo*: initiation-promotion model. *Anticancer Research* 19:3749-3752, 1999.

Iqbal, T. H., Lewis, K. O., and Cooper, B. T.: Phytase activity in human and rat small intestine. *Gut* 35: 1233-1236, 1994.

Jackson, S. P., Bartek, J.: The DNA-damage response in human biology and disease. *Nature* 461: 1071-1078, 2009.

Jagadeesh, S., and Banerjee, P. P.: Inositol hexaphosphate represses telomerase activity and translocates TERT from the nucleus in mouse and human prostate cancer cells via the deactivation of Akt and PKC alpha. *Biochemical & Biophysical Research Communications* 349:1361-1367, 2006.

Jain, P., Nihill, P., Sobkowski, J., Augustin, M.Z.: Commercial soft drinks: pH and *in vitro* dissolution of enamel. *General Dentistry* 55: 150-154, 2007.

Janus, S. C., Weurtz, B., and Ondrey, F. G.: Inositol hexaphosphate and paclitaxel: symbiotic treatment of oral cavity squamous cell carcinoma. *Laryngoscope* 117:1381-1388, 2007.

Jariwalla R. J., Lawson, S., Sabin, R., Bloch, D. A., Prender, M., Andrews, V., and Herman, Z. S.: Effects of dietary phytic acid (phytate) on the incidence and growth rate of tumors promoted in Fisher rats by a magnesium supplement. *Nutrition Res* 8: 813-827, 1988.

Jariwalla R. J., Sabin, R., Lawson, S., and Herman, Z. S.: Lowering of serum cholesterol and triglycerides and modulations by dietary phytate. *J Appl Nutr* 42: 18-28, 1990.

Jariwalla, R. J.: Inositol hexaphosphate (IP6) as an anti-neoplastic and lipid-lowering agent. *Anticancer Research* 19:3699-3702, 1999.

Jenab, M., and Thompson, L. U.: Phytic acid in wheat bran affects colon morphology, cell differentiation and apoptosis. *Carcinogenesis* 21:1547-1552, 2000.

Ji, H., Sandberg, K., Baukal, A. J., and Catt, K. J.: Metabolism of inositol pentakisphosphate to inositol hexakisphosphate in Xenopus laevis oocytes. *Journal of Biological Chemistry* 264: 20185-20188, 1989.

Johnson M, Tucci, M., Benghuzzi, H., Cason, Z., Hughes, J.: The effects of inositol hexaphosphate on the inflammatory response in transformed RAW 264.7 macrophages" in *Biomedical Sciences Instrumentation*. 36: 21-26, 2002.

Juricic J, Druzijanic, N., Perko, Z., Kraljevic, D., and Ilic, N.: IP6 + Inositol in treatment of ductal invasive breast carcinoma: Our clinical experience. *Anticancer Research* 24, 3475, 2004.

Kamp, D. W., Israbian, V. A., Yeldandi, A. V., *et al.*: Phytic acid, an iron chelator, attenuates pulmonary inflammati-on and fibrosis in rats after intratracheal instillation of asbestos. *Toxicologic Pathology* 23:689-695, 1995.

Kamp, D.W., Panduri, V., Weitzman, S. A., and Chandel, N. Asbestos-induced alveolar epithelial cell apoptosis: role of mitochondrial dysfunction caused by iron-derived free radicals. *Mol. Cell. Biochem.* 235: 153-160, 2002.

Kapral M, Parfiniewicz, B., Strzałka-Mrozik B, Zachacz A, Węglarz L. Evaluation of the expression of transcriptional factor NF-κB induced by phytic acid in colon cancer cells. *Acta Pol Pharm.*:697-702, 2008.

Karmakar, S., Banik, N. L., and Ray, S. K.: Molecular mechanism of inositol hexaphosphate-mediated apoptosis in human malignant glioblastoma T98G cells. *Neurochem. Research* 32:2094-2102, 2007.

Karsenty, G., and Ferron, M.: The contribution of bone to whole-organism physiology. *Nature* 481: 314-320, 2012.

Khatiwada, J., Verghese, M., Davis, S., and Williams, L. L.: Green tea, phytic acid and inositol in combination reduced the incidence of azoxymethane-induced colon tumors in Fischer 344 male rats. *J Med Food.* 18 April 18, 2011 [Epub ahead of print].

Kinrys, G., Coleman, E., Rothstein, E.: Natural remedies for anxiety disorders: potential use and clinical applications *Depress Anxiety* 26(3):259-265, 2009.

Kolappaswamy, K., Williams, K. A., Benazzi, C., Sarli, G., McLeod, C. G. Jr., Vucenik, I., De Tolla, L. J.: Effect of inositol hexaphosphate on the development of UVB-induced skin tumors in SKH1 hairless mice. *Comparative Medicine* 59: 147-152, 2009.

Kozuka, S., Nogaki, M., Ozeki, T., and Masumori, S.: Premalignancy of the mucosal polyp in the large intestine: II. Estimation of the periods required for malignant transformation of mucosal polyps. *Dis Colon Rectum* 18: 495-500, 1975.

Kumar, S., M., Reddy, S., Babu, K,. Bhilegaonkar P. M., Shirwaikar, A, and Unnikrishnan, M. K.: Anti-inflammatory and antiulcer activities of phytic acid in rats. *Indian J of Exp. Biol.* 42:179-185, 2004.

Lam, S., McWilliams, A., LeRiche, J., MacAulay, C., Wattenberg, L., Szabo, E. A phase I study of myo-inositol for lung cancer chemoprevention. *Cancer Epidemiol. Biomark. Preven.*15:1526-31, 2006.

Larsson, O., Barker, C. J., Sjoholm, A., *et al*.: Inhibition of phosphatases and increased Ca2+ channel activity by inositol hexa-kisphosphate. *Science* 278:471-474, 1997.

Larsson, S. C., Giovannucci, E., Bergkvist, L., and Wolk, A.: Whole grain consumption and risk of colo-rectal cancer: a population-based cohort of 60,000 women. *British Journal of Cancer* 92:1803-1807, 2005.

Lee, H. J., Lee, S. A., and Choi, H.: Dietary administration of inositol and/or inositol-6-phosphate pre-vents chemically-induced rat hepatocarcinogenesis. *Asian Pacific J of Cancer Prevent.:* 6:41-47, 2005.

Lee, H., Jeong, C., Ghafoor, K., Cho, S., and Park, J.: Oral delivery of insulin using chitosan capsules cross-linked with phytic acid. *Bio-Medical Materials & Engineering* 21: 25-36, 2011.

Lehtihet, M., Honkanen, R. E., and Sjöholm, A.: Inositol hexakisphosphate and sulfonylureas regulate beta-cell protein phosphatases. *Biochemical & Biophysical Res. Communication.* 316: 893-897, 2004.

Li, X., Dai, X., and He, A.: Lung cancer screening in China [T antigen test of sputum – a new simple method for screening lung cancer] in Chinese *Zhonghua Jie He He Hu Xi Za Zhi.* 18 (5): 285-286, 1995.

López-González, A. A., Grases, F., Roca, P., *et al.*: Phytate (*myo*-inositol hexaphosphate) and risk factors for osteoporosis, *J Med Food* 11: 747-752, 2008.

Lord, C. J., and Ashworth, A.: The DNA damage response and cancer therapy. *Nature* 481: 287-294, 2012.

Lott, J. N. A., and Batten, G. G.: Mechanisms and regulation of mineral nutrient storage during seed development. In *Seed Development and Germination*: Kigel, Galili, Eds. Marcel Dekker, New York, pp. 215-235, 1995.

Ma, Y., and Lieber, M. R.: Binding of inositol hexakisphosphate (IP6) to Ku but not to DNA-PKcs. *Journal of Biological Chemistry* 277:10756-10759, 2002.

Macbeth, M. R., Schubert, H. L., Vandemark, A. P., Lingam, A. T., Hill, C. P., and Bass, B. L.: Inositol hexakisphosphate is bound in the ADAR2 core and required for RNA editing. *Science* 309:1534-1539. 2005.

Maffucci, T., Piccolo, E., Cumashi, A., *et al.*: Inhibition of the phosphatadylinositol 3-kinase/Akt pathway by inositol pentakisphos-phate results in anti-angiogenic and antitumor effects. *Cancer Research* 65:8339-8349, 2005.

Malhotra, S. L.: Geographical distribution of gastrointestinal cancers in India with special reference to causation. *Gut* 8:361-372, 1967.

Marks, G., Aydos, R. D., Fagundes, D. J., Pontes,E. R., Takita, L. C., Amaral, E. G., Rossini, A., and Ynouye, C. M.: Modulation of transforming growth factor beta 2 (TGF beta2) by inositol hexaphosphate in colon carcinogenesis in rats. *Acta Cir Bras* 21(supplement 4): 51-56, 2006.

Matejuk, A., and Shamsuddin, A. M.: IP₆ in cancer therapy: Past, present and future. *Current Cancer Therapy Reviews* 6: 1-12, 2010.

McFadden, D. W., Riggs, D. R, Jackson, B. J., and Cunningham, C.: Corn-derived carbohydrate inositol hexaphosphate inhibits Barrett's adenocarcinoma growth by pro-apoptotic mechanisms. *Oncology Reports* 19:563-566, 2008.

McLaurin, J., Golomb, R., Jurewicz, A., Antel, J. P., Fraser, P. E. Inositol stereoisomers stabilize an oligomeric aggregate of Alzheimer amyloid β peptide and inhibit Aβ-induced toxicity. *J Biol Chem.* 275(24): 18495-18502, 2000.

McMillan, B., Riggs, D. R., Jackson, B. J., Cunningham, C., and McFadden, D. W.: Dietary influence on pancreatic cancer growth by catechin and inositol hexaphosphate. *Journal of Surgical Research* 141:115-119, 2007.

Menniti, F. S., Oliver, K. G., Putney, Jr. J. W., and Shears, S. B.: Inositol phosphates and cell signal-ing: new views of InsP5 and InsP6. *Trends in Biochemical Sciences* 18:53-56, 1993.

Miller, J., Cox, G., Radford, K., Zawydiwski, R., and Evelegh, M.: Clinical evaluation of a new screen-ing test for lung cancer based on galactose oxidase-Schiff's reactivity in sputum samples. Presented at the 2003 *Annual Meeting of the American Associa-tion of Cancer Research*. 2003.

Montpetit, B., Thomsen, N.D., Helmke, K.J., Seeliger, M.A., Berger, J.M., and Weis, K.: A conserved mechanism of DEAD-box ATPase activation by nucleoporins and InsP6 in mRNA export. *Nature* e-publication March 27, 2011.

Morrison, R. S., Shi, E., Kan, M., Yamaguchi, F., McKeehan, W., Rudnicka-Nawrot, M., and Palczewski, K.: Inositol hexakisphosphate (InsP6): an antagonist of fibroblast growth factor receptor binding and activity. *In Vitro Cellular & Developmental Biology. Animal* 30A:783-789, 1994.

Morton, R. K., Raison, J. K. A complete intracellular unit for incorporation of amino-acid into storage protein utilizing adenosine triphosphate generated from phytate. *Nature* 200: 429-433, 1963.

Mukherjee, S.: *The Emperor of All Maladies, A Biography of Cancer*. Scribner, New York, 2010.

Muraoka, S., and Miura, T.: Inhibition of xanthine oxidase by phytic acid and its antioxidative action. *Life Sciences* 74:1691-1700, 2004.

Muto, T., Bussey, H. J., and Morson, B.C.: The evolution of the cancer of the colon and rectum. *Cancer* 36:2251-2270, 1975.

Nagata, E., Luo, H. R., Saiardi, A., Bae, B. I., Suzuki, N., and Snyder, S. H.: Inositol hexakisphosphate kinase-2, a physiologic mediator of cell death. *Journal of Biological Chemistry* 280:1634-1640, 2005.

Nahapetian, A., and Young, V. R.: Metabolism of 14C-phytate in rats: effect of low and high dietary calcium intakes. *Journal of Nutrition* 110:1458-1472, 1980.

Nascimento, N. R., Lessa, L. M., Kerntopf, M. R., Sousa, C. M., Alves, R. S., Queiroz, M. G., Price, J., Heimark, D. B., Larner, J., Du, X., Brownlee, M., Gow, A., Davis, C., and Fonteles, M. C.: Inositols prevent and reverse endothelial dysfunction in diabetic rat and rabbit vasculature metabolically and by scavenging superoxide. *Proc National Acad Sci USA* 103:218-223, 2006.

Nelson, R. L., Yoo, S. J., Tanure, J. C., Andrianopoulos, G., and Misumi, A.: The effect of iron on experimental colorectal carcinogenesis. *Anticancer Research* 9:1477-1482, 1989.

Nickel, K. P., and Belury, M. A.: Inositol Hexaphosphate reduces 12-O-tetradecanoylphorbol-13-acetate-induced ornithine decarboxylase independent of protein kinase C isoform expression in keratinocytes. *Cancer Letters* 140:105-111, 1999.

Obata, T.: Phytic acid suppresses 1-methyl-4-phenylpyridinium iron-induced hydroxyl radical generation in rat striatum. *Brain Research* 978:241-244, 2003.

O'Callaghan, T.: The prevention agenda. *Nature* 471: S2-S4, 24 March 2011.

O'Dell, B. L.: Dietary factors that affect biological availability of trace elements. *Annals of the New York Academy of Sciences* 199:70-81, 1972.

Ohkawa, T., Ebusino, S., Kitagawa, M., Morimoto, S., Miyazaki, Y., Yasukawa, S.: Rice bran treatment for patients with hypercalciuric stones: experimental and clinical studies. *Journal of Urology* 132: 1140-1145, 1984.

Palatnik, A., Frolov, K., Fux, M., Benjamin, J.: Double-blind, controlled, crossover trial of inositol versus fluvoxamine for the treatment of panic disorder. *J Clin Psychopharm* 21:335–339, 2001.

Panlasigui, L. N., Thompson, L. U: Blood glucose lowering effects of brown rice in normal and diabetic subjects. *Int J Food Sci Nutr* 57:151-158, 2006.

Pederson, T.: On cancer and people. *Science* 332: 423, 2011.

Peters, U., Sinha, R., Chatterjee, N., Subar, A. F., Ziegler, R. G., Kulldorff, M., Bresalier, R., Weissfeld, J. L., Flood, A., Schatzkin, A., Hayes, R. B., and Prostate, lung, colorectal and ovarian cancer screening trial project team. Dietary fibre and colorectal adenoma in a colorectal cancer early detection programme. *Lancet* 361:1491-1495, 2003.

Phillippy, B.Q., Ullah, A.H., Ehrlich, K.C. Purification and some properties of inositol 1,3,4,5,6-Pentakis-phosphate 2-kinase from immature soybean seeds. *J Biol Chem* 269:28393-28399, 1994.

Porres, J. M., Stahl, C. H., Cheng, *et al*.: Dietary intrinsic phytate protects colon from lipid peroxidation in pigs with a moderately high dietary iron intake. *Proc Soc for Exper Biol & Med* 221:80-86, 1999.

Pretlow, T. P., O'Riordan, M. A., Somich, G. A., Amini, S. B., and Pretlow, T. G.: Aberrant crypts correlate with tumor incidence in F344 rats treated with azoxymethane and phytate. *Carcinogenesis* 13: 1509-1512, 1992.

Ra Yoon M, Hyun Nam, S., Young Kang M.: Antioxidative and antimutagenic activities of 70% ethanolic extracts from four fungal mycelia-fermented specialty rices. *J Clin Biochem Nutr.*118-25, 2008.

Rafacz-Livingston KA, Martinez-Amezcua C, Parsons CM, Baker DH, and Snow J: Citric acid improves phytate phosphorus utilization in crossbred and commercial broiler chicks. *Poult Sci* 84: 1370-1375, 1999.

Raina, K., S. Rajamanickam, R. P. Singh, and R. Agarwal. Chemopreventive efficacy of inositol hexaphosphate against prostate tumor growth and progression in TRAMP mice. *Clinical Cancer Research* 14:3177-3184, 2008.

Rao, P. S., Liu, X. K., Das, D. K., Weinstein, G. S., and Tyras, D. H.: Protection of ischemic heart from reperfusion injury by myo-inositol hexaphosphate, a natural antioxidant. *Annals of Thoracic Surgery* 52:908-912, 1991.

Reddy, N. R., Sathe, S. K., and Salunkhe, D. K.: Phytates in legumes and cereals. *Advances in Food Research* 28:1-92, 1982.

Reece, E. A., Eriksson, U. J.: The pathogenesis of diabetes-associated congenital malformations. *Obstetrics & Gynecology Clinics of North Am* 23: 29-43, 1996

Reece, E. A., Wu, Y-K: Prevention of diabetic embryopathy in offspring of diabetic rats with use of a cocktail of deficient substrates and an antioxidant. *Am J Obstetrics & Gynecology* 176, 790-798, 1997.

Rizvi, I., Riggs, D. R., Jackson, B. J., Ng, A., Cunningham, C., and McFadden, D. W.: Inositol hexaphosphate (IP6) inhibits cellular proliferation in melanoma. *J of Surg Res* 133:3-6, 2006.

Rose, D. P. Dietary fiber and breast cancer. *Nutrition & Cancer* 13:1-8, 1990.

Roy, S., Gu, M., Ramasamy, K., Singh, R. P., Agarwal, C., Siriwardana, S., Sclafani, R. A., and Agarwal, R.: p21/Cip1 and p27/Kip1 Are essential molecular targets of inositol hexaphosphate for its antitumor efficacy against prostate cancer. *Cancer Res.* 1166-73, 2009.

Roy, S., Singh, R. P., Agarwal, C., Siriwardana, S.,. Sclafani, R., and Agarwal, R.: Downregulation of both p21/Cip1 and p27/Kip1 produces a more aggressive prostate cancer phenotype. *Cell Cycle* 7:1828-1835, 2008.

Sakamoto, K., Nakano, G., and Nagamachi, Y.: A pilot study on the usefulness of a new test for mass screening of colorectal cancer in Japan. *Gastro-enterologia Japonica* 25: 432-436, 1990.

Sakamoto, K., Nakano, G., and Nagamachi, Y.: Evaluation of a new test for colorectal neoplasms: A prospective study of asymptomatic population. *Cancer Biotherapy*. 8:49-55, 1993.

Sakamoto, K., Venkatraman, G., and Shamsuddin, A. M.: Growth inhibition and differentiation of HT-29 cells in vitro by inositol hexaphosphate (phytic acid). *Carcinogenesis* 14:1815-1819, 1993.

Sakamoto, K., Vucenik, I., and Shamsuddin, A. M.: [3H]-phytic acid (inositol hexaphosphate) is absorbed and distributed to various tissues in rats. *Journal of Nutrition* 123:713-720, 1993.

Sakamoto. K.: Long-term survival of a patient with advanced non-small cell lung cancer treated with Inositol Hexaphosphate (IP6) plus Inositol treat-ment combined with chemo-radiotherapy. Report of a case. *Anticancer Res* 24, 3618, 2004.

Sakamoto, K., and Suzuki, Y. IP6 plus Inositol treatment after surgery and post-operative radiotherapy. Report of a case: Breast cancer. *Anticancer Res* 24, 3617, 2004.

Sasakawa, N., Sharif, M., and Hanley, M. R.: Metabolism and biological activities of inositol pentakisphosphate and inositol hexakisphosphate. *Biochemical Pharmacology* 50:137-146, 1995.

Saw, N. K., Chow, K., Rao, P. N., Kavanagh, J. P.: Effects of inositol hexaphosphate (phytate) on calcium binding, calcium oxalate crystallization and *in vitro* stone growth.

Schafer, Z. T., Grassian, A. R., Song, L., Jiang, Z., Gerhart-Hines, Z., Irie, H. Y., Gao, S., Puigserver, P., and Brugge, J. S.:Antioxidant and oncogene rescue of metabolic defects caused by loss of matrix attachment. *Nature*. 461(7260):109-13, 2009.

Scherer. Ueber eine neue, aus dem Muskelfleische gewonnene Zuckerart. *Liebigs Ann Chem* 73:322-328, 1850.

Schneider, J. G., Alosi, J. A., McDonald, D. E., and McFadden, D. W.: Effect of pterostilbene on melanoma alone and in synergy with inositol hexaphosphate. *American J Surgery* 198: 679-684, 2009.

Schröterová, L., Hasková, P., Rudolf, E., and Cervinka, M: Effect of phytic acid and inositol on the proliferation and apoptosis of cells derived from colorectal carcinoma. *Oncology Reports* 23: 787-793, 2010

Seeds, A. M., Bastidas, R. J., and York, J. D.: Molecular definition of a novel inositol polyphosphate metabolic pathway initiated by inositol 1,4,5-trisphosphate 3-kinase activity in Saccharomyces cerevisiae. *Journal of Biological Chemistry* 280:27654-27661, 2005.

Shamsuddin, A.K.M., Bell, H.G., Petrucci, J.V., and Trump, B.F.: Carcinoma *in situ* and 'microinvasive' adenocarcinoma of colon. *Pathology Research and Practice*, 167: 374-379, 1980.

Shamsuddin, A.M., Kato, Y., Kunishima, N., Sugano, H., and Trump, B.F.: Carcinoma *in situ* in flat mucosa of large intestine. Report of a case with significance in strategies for early detection. *Cancer* 56: 2849-2854, 1985

Shamsuddin, A.K.M.: Perspectives on large intestinal cancer: Animal models and human disease. *Human Pathology* 17: 451-453, 1986.

Shamsuddin, A., and Elsayed, A.: Hemagglutination inhibition assay for detection of large intestinal cancer associated glycoconjugates in rectal mucus. *Laboratory Investigation* 56: 72A, 1987.

Shamsuddin, A.M., and Elsayed, A.M.: A test for detection of colorectal cancer. *Human Pathology* 19: 7-10, 1988.

Shamsuddin, A.M., Elsayed, A.M., and Ullah, A.: Suppression of large intestinal cancer in F-344 rats by inositol hexaphosphate. *Carcinogenesis* 9: 577-580, 1988.

Shamsuddin, A.M., and Ullah, A.: Inositol hexaphos-phate inhibits large intestinal cancer in F344 rats 5 months following induction by azoxymethane. *Carcinogenesis* 10: 625-626, 1989.

Shamsuddin, A.M., Ullah, A., and Chakravarthy, A.K.: Inositol and inositol hexaphosphate suppress cell proliferation and tumor formation in CD-1 mice. *Carcinogenesis* 10: 1461-1463, 1989.

Shamsuddin, A. M., Elsayed, A. M., and Jockle, G.: Screening Test for Large Intestinal Cancer, U.S. Patent 4, 857, 457. 1989

Shamsuddin, A. M.: Diagnostic Assays for Colon Cancer. *CRC Press*, Boca Raton, FL.1991.

Shamsuddin, A. M., Baten, A., and Lalwani, N. D.: Effects of inositol hexaphosphate on growth and differentiation in K-562 erythroleukemia cell line. *Cancer Letters* 64:195-202, 1992.

Shamsuddin, A. M.: Reduction of Cell Proliferation and Enhancement of NK-Cell Activity, U.S. Patent # 5,082,833. 1992

Shamsuddin, A. M: Rectal Mucus Test and Kit for Detecting Cancerous and Precancerous conditions, U.S.
Patent #5,162,202. 1992

Shamsuddin, A. M: Screening Test and Kit for Cancerous
and Precancerous conditions, U.S. Patent #5, 348,
860.1994.

Shamsuddin, A.M., and Beasley, W.M.: Expression of the
tumor marker D-galactose-ß-[1→3]-*N*-acetyl-D-
galactosamine by premalignant and malignant
prostate. *Arch Pathol & Lab Med* 118: 48-51, 1994.

Shamsuddin, A. M., and G. Y. Yang.: Inositol hexaphosphate inhibits growth and induces differentiation of
PC-3 human prostate cancer cells. *Carcinogenesis*
16:1975-1979, 1995.

Shamsuddin, A.M., Tyner, G.T., and Yang, G.Y.: Common expression of the tumor marker D-galactose-
ß-[1→3]-*N* acetyl-D-galactosamine by different
adenocarcinomas: Evidence of field-effect phenomenon. *Cancer Research* 55: 149-152, 1995.

Shamsuddin, A. M.: Inositol phosphates have novel
anticancer function. *Journal of Nutrition* 125:
725S-732S, 1995.

Shamsuddin, A. M.: A simple mucus test for cancer
screening. *Anticancer Research* 16: 2193-2200,
1996.

Shamsuddin, A. M., Yang, G-Y., and Vucenik, I: Novel anti-cancer functions of IP₆: Growth inhibition and differentiation of human mammary cancer cell lines *in vitro. Anticancer Research* 16: 3287-3292, 1996.

Shamsuddin, A. M., Yang, G. Y., and Vucenik, I.: Novel anti-cancer functions of IP6: growth inhibition and differentiation of human mammary cancer cell lines in vitro. *Anticancer Research* 16:3287-3292, 1996.

Shamsuddin, A. M., Vucenik, I., and Cole, K. E.: IP₆: a novel anti-cancer agent. *Life Sciences* 61: 343-354, 1997.

Shamsuddin, A. M.: Metabolism and cellular functions of IP₆: a review. *Anticancer Res* 19:3733-3736, 1999.

Shamsuddin, A. M., and Vucenik, I.: Mammary tumor inhibition by IP₆ *Anticancer Research* 19: 3671-3674, 1999

Shamsuddin, A. M.: Anticancer function of phytic acid. *International Journal of Food Science and Technology* 37: 769-782, 2002

Shamsuddin, A.: Cell signaling properties of inositol hexaphosphate. In: *Nutrigenomics: The Role of Oxidants and Antioxidants in Gene Expression.* Rimbach G and Packer L, editors. New York, NY, Marcel Dekker Inc., pp 397-420, 2005.

Shamsuddin, A. M., and Vucenik, I.: IP₆ & Inositol in cancer prevention and therapy. *Current Cancer Therapy Reviews* 1:259-269, 2005.

Shamsuddin, A. M, and Vucenik, I.: Prevention of Nuclear, Solar and Other Radiation-Induced Tissue Damage. *US Patent Application* # 11/453,843. 2006.

Shamsuddin, A. M., and von Fraunhofer, J. A.: Reduction of the titratable acidity and the prevention of tooth and other bone degeneration. *US Patent Application* # 11/712,512, 2007.

Sharma, G., Singh, R.P., Agarwal, R.: Growth inhibitory and apoptotic effects of inositol hexaphosphate in transgenic adenocarcinoma of mouse prostate (TRAMP-C1) cells. *Int J Oncol* 23(5):1413-1418, 2003.

Shears, S. B. Inositol pentakis- and hexakisphosphate metabolism adds versatility to the actions of inositol polyphosphates. Novel effects on ion channels and protein traffic. *Sub-Cellular Biochemistry* 26:187-226, 1996.

Shimazawa, M., Watanabe, S., Kondo, K., Hara, H, Nakashima, M., Umemura, K.: Neutrophil accumulation promotes intimal hyperplasia after photochemically induced arterial injury in mice. *European J Pharmacology* 520: 156-163, 2005.

Shivapurkar, N., Tang, Z. C., Frost, A., and Alabaster, O.: A rapid dual organ rat carcinogenesis bioassay for evaluating the chemoprevention of breast and colon cancer. *Cancer Letters* 100:169-179, 1996.

Singh, A., Singh, S. P., and Bamezai, R.: Modulatory influence of arecoline on the phytic acid-altered hepatic biotransformation system enzymes, sulf-hydryl content and lipid peroxidation in a murine system. *Cancer Letters* 117:1-6, 1997.

Singh, R.P., Agarwal, C., and Agarwal, R.: Inositol hexaphosphate inhibits growth, and induces G1 arrest and apoptotic death of prostate carcinoma DU145 cells: modulation of CDKI-CDK-cyclin and pRb-related protein-E2F complexes. *Carcinogenesis* 24:555-563, 2003.

Singh, R. P., Sharma, G., Mallikarjuna, G. U., Dhana-lakshmi, S., Agarwal, C., and Agarwal, R.: *In vivo* suppression of hormone-refractory prostate cancer growth by inositol hexaphosphate: induct-ion of insulin-like growth factor binding protein-3 and inhibition of vascular endothelial growth factor. *Clinical Cancer Research* 10:244-250, 2004.

Slavin, J.: Why whole grains are protective: biological mechanisms. *Proc Nutrition Society* 62:129-134, 2003

Solyakov, L., Cain, K., Tracey, B. M., Jukes, R., Riley, A. M., Potter, B. V., and Tobin, A. B.: Regulation of casein kinase-2 (CK2) activity by inositol phosphates. *Journal of Biological Chemistry* 279:43403-43410, 2004.

Somasundar, P., Riggs, D. R., Jackson, B. J., Cunningham, C., Vona-Davis, L., and McFadden, D. W.: Inositol hexaphosphate (IP6): a novel treatment for pancreatic cancer. *Journal of Surgical Research* 126:199-203, 2005.

Tantivejkul, K., Vucenik, I., Eiseman, J., and Shamsuddin, A. M.: Inositol hexaphosphate (IP₆) enhances the anti-proliferative effects of adriamycin and tamoxifen in breast cancer. *Breast Cancer Research & Treatment* 79:301-312, 2003a.

Tantivejkul, K., Vucenik, I., and Shamsuddin, A. M.: Inositol hexaphosphate (IP₆) inhibits key events of cancer metastasis: I. In vitro studies of adhesion, migration and invasion of MDA-MB 231 human breast cancer cells. *Anticancer Research* 23:3671-3679, 2003b.

Tantivejkul, K., Vucenik, I., and Shamsuddin, A. M.: Inositol hexaphosphate (IP₆) inhibits key events of cancer metastasis: II. Effects on integrins and focal adhesions. *Anticancer Research* 23:3681-3689, 2003c.

Thompson, L. U., and Zhang, L.: Phytic acid and minerals: effect on early markers of risk for mammary and colon carcinogenesis. *Carcinogenesis* 12: 2041-2045, 1991.

Tran, H. C., Gadwal, B. J., Bryant, S, Shamsuddin, A. M., Lunardi-Iskandar, Y., and Vucenik, I.: Effect of inositol hexaphosphate (IP6) on AIDS neoplastic Kaposi's sarcoma, iatrogenic Kaposi's sarcoma and lymphoma. *Proc Am Assoc for Cancer Research* 44: 577-578, Abstract #2536, 2003.

Ullah, A., and Shamsuddin, A.M.: Dose-dependent inhibition of large intestinal cancer by inositol hexaphosphate in F-344 rats. *Carcinogenesis* 11: 2219-2222, 1990.

Vcev, A., Pospihalj, B., Bozic, D., Candrlic, I., Vegar, A., Pinotic, I., and Krucaj, Z.: The galactose oxidase test for detection of colorectal cancer. *Experimental & Clinical Gastroenterology* 1: 217-220, 1991

von Fraunhofer, J. A., Rogers, M. M.: Dissolution of dental enamel in soft drinks. *General Dentistry* pages 308-312, 2004

Vucenik, I., Tomazic, V. J., Fabian, D., and Shamsuddin, A. M.: Antitumor activity of phytic acid (inositol hexaphosphate) in murine transplanted and metastatic fibrosarcoma, a pilot study. *Cancer Letters* 65:9-13, 1992.

Vucenik, I., Sakamoto, K., Bansal, M., and Shamsuddin, A. M.: Inhibition of rat mammary carcinogenesis by inositol hexaphosphate (phytic acid). A pilot study. *Cancer Letters* 75:95-102, 1993.

Vucenik, I., Yang, G. Y., and Shamsuddin, A. M.: Ino-sitol hexaphosphate and inositol inhibit DMBA-induced rat mammary cancer. *Carcinogenesis* 16:1055-1058, 1995.

Vucenik, I., and Shamsuddin, A. M.: [3H]-inositol hexa-phosphate (phytic acid) is rapidly absorbed and metabolized by murine and human malignant cells in vitro. *Journal of Nutrition* 124:861-868, 1994.

Vucenik, I., Yang, G-Y., and Shamsuddin, A.M.: Inositol hexaphosphate and inositol inhibits DMBA-indu-ced rat mammary cancer, *Carcinogenesis* 16: 1055-1058, 1995.

Vucenik, I., Kalebic, T., Tantivejkul, K., and Shamsuddin, A. M.: Novel anticancer function of inositol hexaphosphate: inhibition of human rhabdomyo-sarcoma in vitro and in vivo. *Anticancer Research* 18:1377-1384, 1998.

Vucenik, I., Zhang, Z. S., and Shamsuddin, A. M.: IP6 in treatment of liver cancer. II. Intra-tumoral injec-tion of IP₆ regresses pre-existing human liver cancer xenotransplantcd in nude mice. *Anticancer Research* 18:4091-4096, 1998.

Vucenik, I., Tantivejkul, K., Zhang, Z. S., Cole, K. E., Saied, I., and Shamsuddin, A. M.: IP6 in treatment of liver cancer. I. IP6 inhibits growth and reverses transformed phenotype in HepG2 human liver cancer cell line. *Anticancer Research* 18: 4083-4090, 1998.

Vucenik, I., Podczasy, J. J., and Shamsuddin, A. M.: Antiplatelet activity of inositol hexaphosphate (IP6). *Anticancer Research* 19: 3689-3693, 1999.

Vucenik I, Ramkrishna, G., Tantivejkul K, Anderson L, and Ramljak, D.: Inositol hexaphosphate (IP6) differentially modulates the expression of PKCd in MCF-7 and MDA-MB 231 cells. *Proc Amer Assoc Cancer Res* 40: 653, 1999.

Vucenik, I., Gotovac, J., Druzijanic, N., and Shamsuddin, A.M.: Usefulness of galactose oxidase-Schiff test in rectal mucus for screening of colorectal malignancy. *Anticancer Research.* 21: 1247-1256, 2001

Vucenik, I., and Shamsuddin, A.M.: Cancer Inhibition by inositol hexaphosphate (IP6) and inositol: From laboratory to clinic. *Journal of Nutrition* 133: 3778S-3784S, 2003.

Vucenik, I., Passaniti, A., Vitolo, M. I., Tantivejkul, K., Eggleton, P., and Shamsuddin, A. M.: Anti-angiogenic activity of inositol hexaphosphate (IP6). *Carcinogenesis* 25: 2115-2123, 2004.

Vucenik, I., Ramakrishna, G., Tantivejkul, K., Anderson, L. M., and Ramljak, D.: Inositol hexaphosphate (IP₆) blocks proliferation of human breast cancer cells through a PKCδ-dependent increase in p27Kip1 and decrease in retinoblastoma protein (pRb) phosphorylation *Breast Cancer Research & Treatment* 91: 35-45, 2005.

Vucenik, I., and Ramljak, D.: The contradictory role of PKCδ in cellular signaling. [comment] *Breast Cancer Research & Treatment* 97: 1-2, 2006.

Wattenberg, L. W.: Chemoprevention of pulmonary carcinogenesis by *myo*-inositol. *Anticancer Research* 19: 3659-3661, 1999.

Węglarz, L., Parfiniewicz, B., Orchel, A., and Dzierzewicz, Z.: Anti-proliferative effects of inositol hexaphosphate and verapamil on human colon cancer Caco-2 and HT-29 cells. *Acta Poloniae Pharmaceutica* 63: 443-445, 2006.

Węglarz, L.B., Wawszczyk, J., Orchel, A., Jaworska-kik, M., and Dzierżewicz, Z.: Phytic acid modulates *in vitro* IL-8 and IL-6 from colonic epithelial cells stimulated with LPS and IL-1β. *Digestive Diseases and Sciences* 52: 93-102, 2007.

Weitberg, A.B. A phase I/II trial of beta-(1,3)/(1,6) D-glucan in the treatment of patients with advanced malignancies receiving chemotherapy. *J Exper Clin Cancer Research*. 19: 27-40, 2008.

Williams, K. A., Kolappaswamy, K., De Tolla, L. J., and Vucenik, I.: Protective effect of inositol hexaphosphate against UVB damage in HaCaT cells and skin carcinogenesis in SKH1 hairless mice. *Comparative Medicine* 61: 39-44, 2011.

Winawer, S.J., Zauber, A.G., Ho, M.N. *et al*: Prevention of colorectal cancer by colonoscopic polypectomy. *N Engl J Med* 329: 1977-1981.

Xu, Q., and Reddy, M.B.: Phytic acid protects against 6-OHDA and iron induced apoptosis in cell culture model of Parkinson's disease. *FASEB J* 20: A192. 2006.

Xu Q., Kanthasamy A.G., Reddy M.B.: Neuroprotective effect of natural iron chelator phytic acid in a cell culture model Parkinson's disease. *Toxicology* 245: 101-108, 2008.

Xu, Q., Kanthasamy, A. G., and Reddy, M. B.: Phytic acid protects against 6-hydroxy dopamine-induced dopaminergic neuron apoptosis in normal and iron excess conditions in a cell culture model. *Parkinson's Disease*. 2011:431068, Published online 7 February 2011.

Yang, G. Y., and Shamsuddin, A. M.: IP6-induced growth inhibition and differentiation of HT-29 human colon cancer cells: involvement of intracellular inositol phosphates. *Anticancer Research* 15: 2479-2487, 1995.

Yang, G-Y., and Shamsuddin, A. M.: Gal-GalNAc: a bio-marker of colon carcinogenesis. *Histology and Histopathology* 11: 801-806, 1996.

York, J. D., Odom, A. R., Murphy, R., Ives, E. B., and Wente, S. R.: A phospholipase C-dependent inositol polyphosphate kinase pathway required for efficient messenger RNA export. *Science* 285:96-100, 1999.

Zhang, Z., Song, Y., and Wang, X-L: Inositol hexaphosphate-induced enhancement of natural killer cell activity correlates with suppression of colon carcinogenesis in rats. *World Journal of Gastroenterology* 11: 5044-5046, 2005.

Zhao, D-Y., Feng, F-C., Zhang Y-L., Li, L-B., Xu, G-L., Wan, T-M., Pan, D-S., Zhao, D., Zhang, Y-C., Li, S-B.: Comparison of Shams' test for rectal mucus to an immunological test for fecal occult blood in large intestinal carcinoma screening. Analysis of a check-up of 6480 asymptomatic subjects. *Chinese Medical Journal* 106: 739-742, 1991.

Zhao, Z. and Reece, E. A.: Experimental mechanisms of diabetic embryopathy and strategies for developing therapeutic interventions. *J Soc Gynecol Invest* 12: 549-557, 2005.

Zi, X., R. P. Singh, and R. Agarwal.: Impairment of erbB1 receptor and fluid-phase endocytosis and associated mitogenic signaling by inositol hexaphosphate in human prostate carcinoma DU145 cells. *Carcinogenesis* 21:2225-2235, 2000.

CPSIA information can be obtained
at www.ICGtesting.com
Printed in the USA
LVHW05s1505220618
581594LV00010B/359/P

9 789843 327086